Deeno's Dream Journeys in the Big Blue Bubble

Deeno's Dream Journeys in the Big Blue Bubble

A Relaxation Programme to Help Children Manage their Emotions

Julia Langensiepen

Illustrated by Gerry Turley

Jessica Kingsley Publishers
London and Philadelphia

First published in 2010
by Jessica Kingsley Publishers
116 Pentonville Road
London N1 9JB, UK
and
400 Market Street, Suite 400
Philadelphia, PA 19106, USA

www.jkp.com

Library of Congress Cataloging in Publication Data

Langensiepen, Julia, 1966-
  Deeno's dream journeys in the big blue bubble : a relaxation programme to help children manage their emotions / Julia Langensiepen ; illustrated by Gerry Turley.
    p. cm.
  ISBN 978-1-84905-039-5 (alk. paper)
  1. Emotions in children--Juvenile literature. 2. Stress in children--Juvenile literature. 3. Stress management for children--Juvenile literature. 4. Relaxation--Juvenile literature. I. Turley, Gerry. II. Title. III. Title: Dream journeys in the big blue bubble.
  BF723.E6L38 2010
  155.4'124--dc22

2009019466

British Library Cataloguing in Publication Data
A CIP catalogue record for this book is available from the British Library

ISBN 978 1 84905 039 5

Printed and bound in Great Britain by
Athenaeum Press, Gateshead, Tyne and Wear

Dedicated to my precious daughter Antonia

Acknowledgements

First of all, I want to thank the fantastic children at the 'Blessing Streams' charity in Bangalore, India, for bringing me back to my creative self.

Second, I have to acknowledge that this book would never have been written without the encouragement of my sister Claudia Konrad to take up the training in Autogenics. A big thank you to her.

I would also like to thank my friends Jessie Schuleri and Stefan Frede for their support and friendship; Dr. Patricia Aden, Sabine Seyffert and Claudia Reeker-Lange for their dedication and commitment to their work using Autogenics with children; Jolanthe Herker and Tina Tondar for their technical support; Sylvia Dodson, my sister Christine Fabian and Anna Hayles for their valuable feedback; Alexander Quayle and Sanju Banerjee for their special support and enthusiasm.

CONTENTS

Part B: Children's Introduction

Part C: The Six-Week Programme

Part D: Resources

Preface

Writing this book has been a real pleasure for me. It gave me the opportunity to share a gift that has changed my own life, making it more meaningful, fulfilling and positive.

I was first presented with this gift when I was 40 years old, at the end of my year of volunteering in India and travelling the world. I had handed in my notice as a teacher and had to rebuild my life. I signed up for a course in dance and movement therapy and then trained in Autogenics, a wonderful relaxation/stress management technique.

I had always been a perfectionist and fairly anxious without consciously being aware of it. I functioned and worked very hard but often without having any connection with my true peaceful core. Running marathons, travelling on my own and dancing through my fears but, most of all, learning how to control anxiety and negative feelings through Autogenics has been a very rewarding change for me.

I began applying Autogenics on a daily basis and soon noticed the difference it made. It gave me a real boost and I felt much calmer and more confident.

This book explains how to use this technique with children. It can be used by parents, teachers, teaching assistants, play-workers, therapists, child-psychologists, family therapists, social work-ers and any other professionals interested in working creatively with children to teach and empower them to cope better with the stresses and strains of modern life.

Individual children and their parent(s), guardians or caregiv-ers can learn the technique together at home. Teachers and pupils can choose to do elements of the six-week programme as part of a whole class routine or during circle time. The book also lends itself to use by professionals and children who work together in small groups or on a one-to-one basis.

Part A is written for the adult who will be helping the child learn the technique. It explains a bit about why relaxation is so important, introduces the technique and explains how to use it, whether as a parent at home, or a teacher or other professional, in a group or one-to-one basis

Parts B and C are written as a resource for the children, but should initially be discussed and read through with them. Part B explains how the magic words and stories work, and how best to use the technique when at home. Part C contains the six-week programme, and a follow up on how to create one's own magic words. As you and the child or the children you are working with become more familiar with the technique, then the idea is that they can read up on sections in Parts B and C and look at the il-lustrations in their own time. This is to enable them to take re-sponsibility for their own well-being and read through the magic words and stories whenever they feel like it.

I suggest you read through Parts B and C on your own first to familiarize yourself with and know the material, the method and the stories before going through it with your child or class.

May reading this book bring you the same enjoyment that writ-ing it has brought to me, and may it bring peace and happiness to the children you are using it with.

Part A

Adults' Introduction

1

WHY CHILDREN NEED RELAXATION

Being a child in the 21st century

Children in the Western developed world are growing up in times of rapid technological change and in an extremely fast-moving and hyper-competitive culture. At school they experience a very academic test-driven curriculum and are expected to cope just fine; this is often not the case.

Childhood depression is on the rise, and more and more children are suffering from stress, anxiety, fear of failure and psychosomatic illnesses.

We have allowed technology and the visual image to become dominant today and it is no surprise that a lot of children experience difficulty in dealing with stillness and concentration. They are constantly bombarded with images and loud sounds through TV, DVDs, video games, iPod, mobile phones, aggressive TV marketing strategies, etc.

It is time to offer children a break and give them effective, practical tools to help them to cope. This is what my book is aimed at. It teaches 'Autogenics', a word that comes from the Greek 'auto' meaning self, and 'genus' meaning produced by. In practical terms, it means that once the children have learnt this technique under adult guidance they will be able to use it independently whenever they need it. It will guide them safely back to a quiet place within and they will be better equipped to deal with their day-to-day challenges. It will give them a tower of strength at their core, a valuable source of peacefulness that they can tap into autonomously at any time.

In an ideal world, children would all learn this relaxation technique before they start showing signs of stress, inability to cope at school and before psychosomatic illnesses start to set in. This way a child could learn the technique unburdened and free of any difficulties. If the school day started with a group relaxation exercise and children knew how to keep their concentration it would make life so much more enjoyable at school for both teachers and students alike.

About the technique

The Autogenic relaxation technique as explained in my book is easy to learn and has been used successfully with children and teenagers since the mid 1970s. It is a highly regarded method in mainland Europe, often recommended or taught by GPs, paediatricians, teachers, therapists and play-workers as a very effective means to prevent and combat stress and stress-related illnesses in children. There is nothing mystical about this training. It's pure physiology. It takes six weeks to learn the exercises which will enable the child to lead a happier, healthier, successful life. The benefits will be felt fairly quickly.

What it is

In the 1930s a well-known Berlin-based neurologist, Dr. J.H. Schultz, developed a special technique to help his clients to relax.

He called it 'Autogenics' and divided it into six basic exercises: 1. Heaviness, 2. Warmth, 3. Breath, 4. Heart, 5. Solar plexus or stomach and 6. Forehead. The learner assumes a comfortable position and gently induces a state of relaxation through silently repeating a series of carefully designed formulae (what I'm calling 'magic words' for the children). These involve the mind and body and create a very soothing effect on the autonomous nervous system.

In this guide, Schultz's exercises have been simplified and adapted creatively to provide a stimulating and fun way to engage children in relaxation.

How it works

When practising an Autogenic exercise, we feel at rest, at peace, in a pleasurable state which is often described as the 'Autogenic state'. It has a profound impact on our physiology because it activates the peaceful part of the autonomous nervous system, which shuts down the stress response and takes control to offer a calm reaction. Thus the heart rate decreases, breathing slows down, muscle tension decreases and all the other flight–fight symptoms are reversed.

In this guide for children I have included illustrations, visualization exercises and creative stories along with the magic words for each week, which the adult takes them through and helps them to understand. This is to make the learning of each of the magic words as easy and fun as possible through appealing to the child's senses and imagination and thus engaging the child at all levels. It will create a pattern in their memory which they will then later be able to access very easily during their own short daily practice.

Then, through the use of the creative stories which incorporate the magic words with elements of guided imagery the children are taken on a health-giving journey. They are asked to close their eyes, lie down or sit still and concentrate on emptying their minds of all emotions and thought in order to concentrate on the images and places to which the story will take them.

Just as we can make negative use of our imagination through constant worrying and worst-case-scenario thoughts that make us tense and nervous, positive use of our imagination has healing powers and the capacity to make us feel calm and re-energized.

In each story, the child is addressed directly which is why he/she feels subconsciously part of it, accompanying the hero, Deeno the dinosaur, to safe, deeply relaxing and wonderful places. The child is encouraged to tap into his/her own creative resources and imagination through the choice of words and suggestive adjectives. Every child can paint his/her own picture and imagine what he or she wants to see during the story; the size of the big blue bubble, where it will take them and so on. All of this allows him/her to remember and recall the calming journey, the peaceful atmosphere and the magic words round which it is all based much more vividly and thus reuse this positive pattern to stay calm in times of stress.

The benefits
General benefits

Over a sustained period of regularly practising this technique the immune system gets stronger and stressful situations can be coped with much better. One generally approaches daily tasks with a more positive and calmer outlook.

Initially, it is best to practise in a silent place, always at the same time to build it into the daily routine. Once this becomes second nature, the body gets programmed to react to the formulae wherever you are and whatever time it is. The auto-response is very strong and efficient. It is a matter of training your body through regular small repetitions. A huge benefit is that people who have been practising the technique for a while are much more in tune with their bodies and receive or acknowledge their body's stress symptoms and signals much quicker. They can use it in almost any situation to instantly recharge their batteries, get a quick release of energy, or to calm down, let go of stress, combat fear and panic. It is thus a very effective and practical tool on your way to a calmer, happier lifestyle. No need for any tapes, CDs or anything else to carry around – the source of strength you are tapping into lies within you.

Benefits for children

For any child, learning this technique will offer a definite improvement to their lifestyle and performance by creating a healthier balance and offering the learning of a new skill. The relaxation technique promotes a greater sense of responsibility, due to the fact that they practise on their own through their own motivation and dedication. It gives them the opportunity to develop their own personality and to gain greater independence though healthy detachment from their parents. Results are generally seen quickly if the children practise regularly and this is very motivating. Agreeing to a minimum of six regular sessions with their parent or an adult to learn the technique and having to set up and stick to their own practice routine teaches children that discipline is necessary if they want to feel better and see changes in themselves. This learning experience creates a skill which they will benefit from forever; they can take it with them and apply it to different areas of their lives. From a mental strength point of view, it equips the child to cope better with adapting to the constantly changing environment and challenges of which life consists.

Autogenic relaxation can be offered to children for a variety of reasons:

1. as a solution to existing stress-related psychosomatic illnesses in children

2. as a preventative measure, to minimize the potential risk of a child's tendency to stress

3. as a pro-active measure to raise children's awareness of healthy options.

No matter at what stage you introduce it, there are many positive effects through learning this relaxation technique for any child including:

- increased confidence

- greater sense of responsibility

- better memory

- improved concentration

- enhanced physical and mental performance

- greater inner strength.

The first sign that a child is reacting positively practising the relaxation technique on a daily basis is usually better quality sleep. Other improvements will follow.

A typical programme session

A typical session of 'the magic words in six weeks' might take the format shown in the box.

SUMMARY OF THE WEEKLY SESSIONS:

1. The week's magic words

   Introduce, explain and learn the new magic words, adding them onto the words from the previous week. Read about what is meant to happen, and the purpose of words. Your aim is for them to understand the physiological explanation about what will happen in their body if they concentrate on the meaning of the words. There are also points for discussion, to further stimulate their thinking around the words and their meaning.

2. Warm-up activities

   The aim is to deepen their understanding of the magic words through creative physical activities including visualizations, movement, getting in touch with nature, and learning breathing techniques, before assuming a comfortable position to do the relaxation exercise and familiarize themselves with the new magic words of the week, whilst listening to a creative story.

3. The week's story

   The magic words for the week are absorbed through a creative story which the adult reads to the child in a very calming voice as part of an evening routine or therapy session, circle time or whole class routine. They follow the main character, Deeno, to a number of very safe, magic, imaginary places. On these journeys, they learn to de-stress, manage their anger and improve concentration. Visualization and affirmation exercises build self-esteem and self-awareness.

4. On their own that week

   In order to properly absorb the week's magic words, it is essential that they practise on their own on a daily basis before adding on the next magic words. They don't need to read the story or do the activities again, just spend a few minutes each day, preferably a few times each day, reciting the magic words silently in their head, and really thinking about what the words mean and imagining the changes that are happening in their bodies as they say them. They are responsible for building these short bursts of time for relaxation into their daily routine. It is a matter of training the body through regular small repetitions; this is how the relaxation response becomes second nature for the children. This will be explained further in Part B under 'Setting up a routine' (see pp.59–60).

5. Follow-up activities

Following the relaxation magic words and story of the week, you could invite the children to comment on the story and perhaps do a follow-up activity, such as creative drawing or writing in a journal. This will help them to digest and remember the new magic words more easily.

NOTE: At the beginning of each session, ask them to briefly summarize and refer back to what they learnt or discussed in the previous session to get them into the subject matter and to clarify any questions or misunderstandings. You can also ask how they got on with their individual practice routine; in what situations they have used the magic words, how it has helped them and, if necessary, give practical tips on how to build in little bursts of magic words practice into their daily routine. If the children do not have their own copy of the book it could be worth your while copying the summary page of all the magic words from the last chapter (see p.120) and give this to the child/children to display in their room.

2

RELAXATION
AT HOME

Being a parent in the 21st century

It has always been a tough job to bring up children. Why? Because it is relentless, 24 hours a day, it never stops. In our fast moving, technological age ruled by globalization it has become even harder. Jobs move families around the globe breaking up the extended family and communities. Jobs are no longer for life, there is high job-insecurity and we are told that to be successful we must be flexible. Our culture is steering us away from traditional family values towards constantly striving to improve our image through greater income and possessions. Striving to pay for a specific lifestyle, the majority of parents feel exhausted and guilty about not having enough time and energy left for parenting. The work/life balance debate is often a very touchy subject and easily ignored in our competitive consumer culture. As parents, however, you know you are your child's main role-model. They will look at how you react in stressful situations and subconsciously copy you. If you want your child to grow into a happy, confident and resilient teenager they need time, love, attention and good role-modelling throughout childhood from the significant adult in their life.

With this book it is my intention to give you the chance of having healthy winding-down time with your child, away from the box, the internet or other more common, modern ways of switching off and introduce them instead to relaxation using a sensitive and creative approach. Just find some time and a quiet place and read the appropriate chapters with your child. You will feel how the day's stress and tension will start to drain away from your child and also, with a little bit of luck, yourself!

Reading the stories to your child

When you are reading out loud to your child it would be a real bonus for the delivery of the relaxation story if you were feeling calm and relaxed yourself before you start. Create a nice atmosphere for you and your child; maybe light a candle or get a few cushions or a cuddly blanket. Get your child to lie down on the floor until they feel really comfortable in the correct practice position and say a few calming sentences to prepare your child before you start reading the story, for instance:

Try to get really comfortable...and when you are feeling that nothing is distracting you any more, close your eyes...feel your body, how it is supported by the floor...and then listen to the story...

It is equally important to end the story with calm, but clear instructions for your child to find her/his way out of the story:

In a few minutes we will have to finish the story and when I tell you to close the exercises I would like you to make a strong fist with both hands... Bend/flex your elbows sharply several times... Open your eyes wide... Take a few deep breaths and have a good stretch.

The beginning and the end of the story should always be the same. This will give your child a feeling of security as they will know what to expect. Should you be reading the story at bedtime, just leave out the end bit about 'closing the exercise' so your child can take the story into their dreams.

Relaxation stories are to be read in a calm, soft voice without haste or hurry. Wherever the magic words appear in the story, they are printed in bold. These should be reinforced through reading them more slowly and lengthening the individual words, giving your child the chance to really feel the physical changes in their body taking place. It is important to leave enough time in between the sentences for your child to be able to follow, imagine and enjoy what is happening in the story. Your voice is the carrier of relaxation and the peaceful images for your child so it is important to watch the speed at which you are reading. Get your child to repeat the magic words quietly in their head as you are reading the story. This will reinforce the physiological changes and it will make sure the child takes an active part in the listening.

Practising

Help your child to create a cosy corner somewhere in your home where you and your child can learn the technique together. During the week, your child can then use the same space for their individual daily practice sessions. A few cushions, a blanket, a candle or an oil burner can add a relaxing touch to a room. Make sure the rest of the family knows what you are doing and respects your quiet time.

Each session is designed to help your child to experience a quiet moment after a busy day. Mood music can be used to enhance the calming effect. However, make sure it is purely instrumental as the lyrics can be distracting.

During the six-week programme, it is advisable to practise saying the magic words as frequently as possible during the day, perhaps two to three times, for about two to three minutes. Once your child masters the individual exercises and can feel the effect physiologically it suffices to practise once a day for about ten minutes. It takes a while for the body to get familiar with the exercises and react to the magic words. It is a gradual process; patience, consistency and trust in the results are vital for it to work.

It makes sense to embed the practising of the Autogenic exercises as a natural component into your child's daily routine. Otherwise, your child will be tempted to procrastinate. It is an enormous help for your child to know that practising the magic words quickly in the morning before school, when coming back from school in the afternoon before watching any television or playing any computer games, and again at night before going to sleep is part of their routine. Practising will then become as normal as having breakfast, washing their hands before eating or brushing their teeth at bedtime.

Once your child is familiar with the technique, it will help them to cope better in stressful situations, and give them access to a truly healthy, happy lifestyle in this fast changing, modern world.

How to best prepare and support your child

Effective leverage

It is vital for your child's success with learning this relaxation technique that you as parents are clear about the reason why you want your child to learn it in the first place. Once you have decided on that, please take the time to talk to your child and make it clear to them what the purpose of learning the technique really is. The success of any learning depends very much on the interest and motivation of the individual participant. The thought of feeling strong and healthy and thus being able to get through homework tasks more swiftly and with better results can prove to be simple but effective leverage and motivation for a child.

Creating a routine during the six-week initial training period

Explain to your child the benefits of learning a relaxation technique with you and what they will gain from it: being less anxious at school, completing their homework much faster, generally being able to concentrate more effectively, sleeping better, etc. Set up a routine and determine a fixed day and time when you meet on a weekly basis to read and work through each part of the book and follow the programme. You might set up a small group with other mums or dads and their children who also want to learn the technique. It will help your child to realize that they are not alone in experiencing certain problems. They will enjoy doing the activities and listening to the stories even more.

The role of siblings

Come to an agreement with the rest of the family that the child concerned is not to be disturbed during relaxation practice and that the place and time they choose is respected and treated as quiet time by any siblings. You can teach the technique to more than one of your children at the same time but they should not be more than two years in age apart.

Putting on the brakes at the right time

Imagine being on a bike going down a steep hill. If you don't use the brakes at regular intervals during the steep descent you will hardly come to a smooth, safe and quick stop at the bottom of the hill. The same applies to your child, if you want to avoid her/him being totally hyper in the evening at bedtime, and unable to calm down and sleep. Have a look at your child's weekly activity plan and ask yourself whether there is enough time built in on a regular daily basis for your son/daughter to 'hibernate' just like any computer does before you switch it off at the end of the working day. Your child needs such quiet times at regular intervals throughout the day to re-charge. In this context, there is the metaphor of the bike I was given during my own training as a relaxation facilitator.

Quality time for relaxation feedback

Give your child the time to talk to you about their experiences with the relaxation technique. Ask about the stories and images that have come up for your child. Emotions can be accessed and tapped into during the relaxation process which might possibly need your time and help. However, be gentle in your approach. Don't force your child to talk to you about the relaxation sessions if they do not need or want to do so. Remember that learning the technique is aimed at lowering the pressure that already exists in their life, not at increasing it.

Quality time leading back to nature

Lead your child away from television and back to nature. Go for walks or bike rides in the park or countryside. Here, your child can learn to re-connect with stillness, with the sounds of birds, with the sound of the wind and with themselves. The fresh air will do your child the world of good. Not only will your child be able to sleep better but they will also take beautiful memories from the day out in nature with them into the land of dreams.

Swapping roles

It might be an interesting change if you let your child teach you the relaxation technique! Swap roles. Why shouldn't your son or daughter read you a relaxing story for a change? It is also a way of acknowledging their efforts and letting them know that you take their relaxation learning very seriously.

How to keep your child motivated

Reminding them of the benefits

If your child is reluctant to practise, remind them of what they are gaining from completing a six-week relaxation programme with you; how the technique will stand them in good stead forever in terms of mental strength, for example getting more swiftly through their homework. Only if your child truly understands why they should be learning the technique will they be willing to keep practising.

Supporting independence

Offer your child your support but refrain from always practising together. After all, this technique aims at making your child an autonomous learner. At the end of the programme they should be able to use this relaxation technique totally independently to cope successfully with stressful situations.

Praise

The most effective way to achieve positive behaviour is to praise good practice. Noticing and complimenting their efforts will make your child feel respected and their self-esteem will grow. You can either say to them what exactly it is you like about their behaviour, what is known as descriptive praise, or else award stickers or little treats to commend positive effort. If your child does not practise, give him a card or a sticker expressing sadness. This could be a sad face printed onto a card and then laminated, which you could place on the fridge next to their practice diary. (Read more about the practice diary in Part B, p.61.) As soon as your child starts to show good behaviour this card can be turned over to the happy face again. If, after a while, your child still does not practise, it will be necessary to have a longer chat.

Being a positive role-model

As a parent, you are your child's number one role-model. Your child looks for patterns of behaviour in you and copies them subconsciously. Reading up on behaviourist theories like those of Albert Bandura or Ivan Pavlov can be fascinating and quite revealing. I have listed some books you might want to read in the Resources section at the back of this book. Think about your own typical response to stress and ways to regain peace and quiet. It might be a real motivator for your child if you took up learning this relaxation technique yourself. You would gain a much better understanding of the learning process your child is going through – it will be a great bonding experience for both of you.

Furthermore, if your child sees you learning this relaxation technique she/he will not be tempted to think she/he has to learn relaxation because he/she is ill or has done something wrong or naughty. She/he will look at you as the role-model and accept this technique as a normal part of a healthy lifestyle.

3

RELAXATION AT SCHOOL

Teaching in the 21st century

As a teacher you have the responsibility to teach children what the national curriculum deems important for our youngsters in order to develop basic numerical and literacy skills. In recent years, the UK government has introduced new measures like circle time and buddy schemes to focus more attention on the social and emotional aspects of learning, which, in theory, is very positive. However, it can be a struggle fitting it all in and without adequate teaching material, instilling these new measures can become ineffectual, disappointing or even destructive.

Teaching under-twelves in the 21st century is complex and not just based on skills learnt at teacher training. You need to develop a great amount of sensitivity to pick up behaviours that demand closer attention. You are the first point of contact for parents when things are not going according to plan with their child. There are an increasing number of children being diagnosed with learning and/or behavioural difficulties and often it is your knowledge and diplomacy that relates these issues from one party to another. Your job as educators is about offering the children a challenging, stimulating and fun learning experience and at the same time creating an atmosphere conducive to their individual learning style. Easier said than done in our modern society, which favours a school system that is so results driven, starts education so early and does not consider the different developmental stages of boys and girls resulting in a lot of boys lagging behind, and feeling inadequate. There are no easy answers as to how to meet all these needs and demands. However, I am convinced that relaxation has to be part of the school day. This won't just help the children, but will also bring great relief to you. It is no quick fix, but after a while you will start to notice how the children in your class have become calmer and more focused on the tasks in hand.

Creating a community for relaxation

This book is a resource that can help to create a community where relaxation is accepted as part of the normal school routine. Building such a community is the most effective way to develop a non-aggressive group ethos where mutual respect, openness and trust prevail.

The following are some ways in which such a community can be built in the classroom or any other group.

Setting realistic goals

As I said before, in order to change the atmosphere in your classroom or the group of children you are working with, and to improve concentration and attitude, regular relaxation sessions are a fantastic initiative that will pay off in the long run. However, if you work with a whole class of over 15 pupils you need to be realistic. This book won't work miracles. If you want to go deep and achieve real results then you will need to work with a smaller group of children, not more than six per session, get them to practise daily on their own and do all the activities. Generally speaking, share your thoughts on why you want to introduce relaxation sessions with the children. It is important that they understand and are comfortable with the idea of relaxing with you.

Time-tabling relaxation

It is necessary to offer the relaxation sessions regularly. Only then will there be positive changes in the children. If you make it part of the weekly plan the children will react very positively as they will be expecting it. However, keep the sessions short and be patient. Initially, some children will find it extremely challenging to sit or lie down quietly for more than five minutes. But after a while they might even start to ask you for extra sessions when they feel tired or tense.

The relaxation can be time-tabled once a week for 10–20 or even 40 minutes. It very much depends on your time availability, group size and age, and what you aim to achieve with the relaxation sessions. Give them a gentle lead-in with shorter sessions at the beginning and gradually extending the time you spend concentrating on the exercises and relaxing together. As you know, every group is different and you need to use your professional judgement as to how quickly or slowly to proceed. Choose a time, however, when both you and the children are fresh and are not feeling under pressure.

The setting

Room size – Ideally, you will have a carpeted area large enough for the children to sit in a circle, engage in moderate movement activities and later on to lie on yoga mats for your relaxation sessions. It needs to be a very quiet space with no-one disturbing or barging in during the session.

A centre piece — Children like it if there is something eye catching like flowers, a candle or an oil burner in the middle of the room. It could also be a symbolic object to represent the magic words of the session. This shows them all that the relaxation session is about to begin, focuses their attention and, if the child is a visual learner, helps them to remember the magic words. However, make sure it is in line with health and safety regulations at your school or the institution/building where you are working.

The atmosphere — Make sure it is calm and cosy and have a sign on the door outside telling others the group are not to be disturbed during the next session. Starting in a circle is ideal if the group is small enough as it is very group-affirming; everyone is part of the group, can see each other and you can establish eye-contact as a way of giving recognition to each child. The children themselves might have a view on the best community setting for their relaxation session. You can work with quiet relaxing background music if you prefer but make sure you listen to it beforehand with your eyes closed. The children must not be distracted by singing voices and the lyrics they are hearing while trying to concentrate on the relaxation story that you are reading to them. The better option is to play them some gentle soft music after the story while they are still dreaming or when they are talking about it, or busily capturing their mind pictures with crayons on paper.

Ensure you have all the equipment needed for the creative activities and that everyone is comfortable in the setting before opening the session with the starting ritual. As I said before, this gives the child(ren) a sense of security and trust and it is vital to create the right atmosphere from the beginning.

Agreed ground rules

As with any group activity with children, agreed rules help to make the relaxation session a success. One way is to write them down and have them on display as a simple reminder during the sessions. Another way is to let the children work in pairs to devise their own rules and then agree democratically on six rules for the whole group. Some ideas are as follows:

- Only the person holding a certain agreed object (tiny dinosaur, ball, magic stone, etc.) is allowed to talk.

- We will listen to each other without interrupting.

- We have the right to pass on the talking object and decide not to talk. We will be given another chance later.

- We all say good things about each other and do not laugh at or ridicule each other.

- There is no talking during the relaxation story.

- We have the right not to close our eyes during the relaxation story but we must cover our eyes with our hands and look down, or if we are lying down, we look at the ceiling, find our favourite spot and fix our gaze during the story. (If the children are sitting at their desks, they can cover their eyes with their hands and put their heads on the table.)

- We have to leave the group and sit out for two minutes if we do not adhere to these rules.

Adult helpers

If you do have adult helpers with you in the relaxation sessions, make sure they sit on the floor with you in the circle. Otherwise it might change the atmosphere and they are seen as intruders rather than helpers. They need to join in all the activities and you ought to point out to them the children who are likely to benefit most from their participation. Next, I will talk about informing the parents as they can prove to be an invaluable source of help for your group.

Informing the parents

Inform the parents about the introduction of relaxation in the class/group: either by just sending a letter out or asking them to come to an info evening at the school. It might be an idea to tell them, first, why you think it is a good idea for children to learn relaxation and, second, what the likely benefits for the children should be. If they come to the school, parents usually react very positively if you read them an imaginative story. They can then understand through their own experience how relaxing and calming such journeys into the world of fantasy creatures and far away places really are. It might also be advisable to recommend that the parents get hold of their own copy of this book. It enables them to support your relaxation work in school with follow-up reading together with their child at home. After a while, you can tell them, their child will be able to use the book independently to help them with their relaxation practice. This is also a good opportunity for you to encourage parents to come along to the relaxation sessions and join in, if it is appropriate in your setting. The parents may gain a lot from joining in. The more adult helpers the better in some schools, but you will need to offer some initial training.

The teacher as role-model

The teacher's role in a relaxation community involving children in an inward-facing activity is a challenging one. I can imagine that some of you think, 'Well, she has not come across a student like such and such or so and so. My pupils couldn't, wouldn't even try to concentrate on relaxation, they are too active, can't expect them to sit still…' As adults we may just see little Harry, the ten-year-old disadvantaged child, or Harry the disruptive boy, and tend to overlook the pure potential of the human spirit, ready to be developed. In the best sense of the word relaxation is a discipline which can be nurtured in everyone. However, you are their role-model, so it is important that you can show that you are able to relax in stressful situations. Children watch the adult who is responsible for them very carefully. If you are keeping calm, relaxed and on top of things on a hectic, busy day your pupils will be much more likely to keep their cool. It might be an idea for you to engage in some sort of relaxation practice for yourself including yoga, Pilates, chanting or Autogenics so you can appreciate the relaxing and calming qualities of such activities.

Regular feedback

Especially in a small group setting, it is important to get regular feedback from the children, how they feel about the sessions and what they think they are getting out of them. It is all too easy for the adult leading the group to get complacent and before they know it, the sessions are boring and repetitive. This applies, in particular, if you want to keep the sessions going after you've completed the Autogenic programme offered in this book. It is important that it remains quality time for you and the group. You can use other stories for relaxation purposes or possibly start to write your own. Make sure you plan the sessions carefully and know the material well in advance.

Follow-up work

Why not talk to your colleagues about relaxation? Maybe they would be interested in doing a whole year project on it. It is always good to spread the word and work on something together. An assembly is another idea to get the whole school informed about this technique.

Whole class relaxation

How effective the technique is will depend on how much time and space you have at your disposal. Teachers working with a whole class and not much time might prefer to leave out the creative activities and just concentrate on learning the magic words and reading the stories that reinforce them. You might also give the children a copy of all the magic words on one page, which you will find towards the end of Part C (p.120). They can then stick it into their homework diaries and highlight each week's magic words as they learn them. They can also use them at night when they go to sleep, or when they are in a stressful situation.

Space should be less of an issue. You don't need any equipment apart from maybe a CD player for soft background music, if you choose to have this. If necessary, the children can just stay seated at their desks and when you read the story, they can close their eyes and put their heads on their desks to avoid distraction. This work won't go as deep but if you do regular sessions at the beginning of the school day, the whole classroom atmosphere amongst the group of children can change and become calmer.

It takes a lot of initiative and energy to introduce relaxation into your school or classroom on a regular basis, especially when time and space can be limited. Be patient. I am sure you will see the benefits of your work. It is a lot of fun to work with children in this way, to take them on imaginary journeys and show them how to access a source of peacefulness that they can tap into at any time.

For other professionals

This section is aimed at paediatricians, play-workers, paediatric nurses, therapists, child-psychologists, family therapists, social workers and any other professionals interested in working creatively with children to teach and empower them to cope better with the stresses and strains of modern life.

From reading through the previous chapters you will have come to realize that this technique is very versatile. It lends itself to use in almost any setting and environment, provided it is quiet, so I am sure you will be able to find a way to adapt it to your specific working conditions.

- It can be very effective used alongside other therapy treatments to further reduce emotional and behavioural problems. It can help you to enable the child or children you are working with to re-gain a sense of happiness at home and at school. As you are well aware, we cannot change a child's environment but we can teach them techniques for how to cope better with stress factors such as sibling rivalry, parental divorce, and change of lifestyle, change of school, violence and arguments in the family. This book can be an additional element in your therapeutic tool bag.

- At specialized children hospitals or psychosomatic clinics, the young patients are dealing with serious illnesses and react with various levels of anxiety. As the age range and the stages at which each young patient is admitted or released vary considerably, it would probably not be possible to take all the children they are working with at any one time through the six-week programme of this book. However, introducing Deeno and his story, the tensing and relaxing section of Part B and covering just weeks one to three are certainly a practical option. Simply knowing and using the first few magic words will have a calming effect on the young patient during his/her hospital stay with all the challenges that may bring. Alternatively, the 12- or 13-year-old patients could benefit from and enjoy reading the stories themselves. The individual play-worker will certainly find new ideas and inspiration through reading this book and can adjust them to his/her own way of working with anxious young patients. They may also encourage parents to use this book at home with their children after the hospital experience. Knowing and using the magic words and being able to transport him/herself away to magic places in the bubble can help a child to regain inner strength and alleviate the burden of having to live with a chronic illness and coming to terms with a serious illness.

- Social workers deal with young individuals facing a huge range of challenges. If they can be taught, no matter where they are, how to create an oasis of peace from which to draw strength from within, it may prevent them from developing serious emotional or behavioural difficulties later on. It is usually a good experience for children to be learning this technique as part of a small group with children of roughly the same age, give or take two years. They tend to learn Autogenics fairly quickly and it will help them to cope with life in a less nurturing environment than they deserve. In the relaxation group they will be able to share their worries and problems and it may well give them consolation that they are not on their own with such challenges. If you teach this technique to the parents separately, they can then choose to continue using it together with their children at home and create a more loving, peaceful rapport with them at bedtime.

I have had very positive reactions from all the children I have worked with. If a child chooses to, this technique can be with them for life and may help them develop into a more assertive, confident person, who is better equipped to deal with life's challenges.

Part B

Children's Introduction

4

THE MAGICAL WORLD
OF RELAXATION

Introduction

Sometimes, there are surely moments and days in your life, when all you want to do is to get as far away from everything as possible; perhaps be all alone on a little island, or maybe drift away into space on a soft white cloud. You would like to get away from school, your parents, siblings, your friends and maybe even leave behind your favourite toy, your dog or cat. You might be feeling tired, exhausted, disappointed, sad, or really annoyed and angry and all you want is some peace and quiet. It could be that your tummy is aching, or your head, and you are feeling restless. You might be anxious because of school and you cannot get to sleep at night because disturbing thoughts are keeping you awake.

No matter what is troubling you, there is a solution. I cannot work magic but I can teach you some magic words that, when repeated to yourself, if you really concentrate on the words and what they mean, will have a magical effect on your health and happiness. You will be lying on a blanket on the floor and you will feel very relaxed. A good way of relaxing is using your imagination, for example concentrating on seeing a big bubble coming your way that takes you to magic places and leads you into a new world. If you like, you can go with Deeno on imaginative journeys to a wild island or deep into the blue sea to the home of the fish, or to the top of a mountain and to lots of other places, where you will feel very calm and safe.

After having heard the magic words and listened to an imaginative story you will be surprised how relaxed you'll feel, how fit and energetic. With regular, short, daily practice of the technique you will see that most of your problems are indeed quite small and you can solve them. School will be fun again, you will get faster at doing your homework and you will feel stronger, healthier and if you happen to argue with your friends it will not bother you as much, as you will know it's not forever and there is a solution if you stay calm.

Deeno's story

Deeno used to be a very sad, lonely dinosaur. He did not have many friends and he always felt that something was wrong with him. When he went out to play he was scared that the other children would laugh at him. He could not concentrate very well in class and was terrified the teacher would call on him to answer a question. Quite often, when he came home from school his mother would pounce on him: 'So,' she would say, 'tell me, Deeno, how was school? What did you do today? Have you eaten all your lunch? Did you get into trouble? How did the maths test go? Who did you play with?' and so she went on and on.

I am sure you can imagine that Deeno did not like coming home after school with such a shower of questions welcoming him at the door. He wished his mother would just let him get on with it, leave him alone.

However, he felt too weak, and did not want to upset her, so he sat down with her in the kitchen and answered each question his mother squeezed out of him and felt deeply unhappy, his hands tightly clenched into fists in his lap until his knuckles went white.

When his headaches became too much and he could not go to sleep any more at night his mother took him to the doctor. He listened very carefully to what was happening and then he said: 'Deeno, it sounds to me like you are a little tense and anxious. How about doing some relaxation exercises? I know a book that may help you. First you read it together with your mother or father to learn the technique properly and then you can do it on your own. It will take you six weeks to master the technique.' Deeno thought it might be worth a try and agreed to do it.

Deeno got home that day, closed the door of his room and opened up the book that the doctor had given him. Inside he found stories about a big blue bubble, a place where he could be comfortable and happy, and some special magic words to recite – a new set of words for each of the six weeks. After the first week of practising the magic words, Deeno began to notice that strange things were happening. The first thing that improved was his sleep. It was amazing how much better he felt in the mornings when waking up. He got to sleep much easier, and woke up ready to attack the day in the morning. Even breakfast tasted better! The second thing that he noticed was that he could concentrate much better once he had done a quick relaxation session. He got through his homework in no time. Then, at school, he noticed his grades began to improve, and he did not mind answering questions in class as much as before. He felt so much happier that he began to play with the other kids more at break time, and to make new friends.

Now when Deeno comes home from school in the afternoon he asks his mother to let him go to his room first. She smiles and lets him go, knowing that he will come down in a few minutes after he has done his relaxation practice and exercises and feels ready to have a little calm chat about his day.

Deeno is not a sad, lonely dinosaur any more. He is so much happier now that he has learnt how to relax with the big blue bubble, and he wants to give you his special book so that you can learn too!

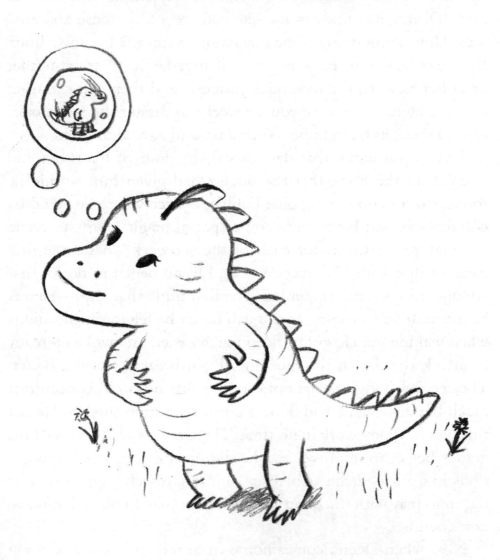

Points for discussion

- How was Deeno feeling at the beginning of the story? Why?

- What did the doctor think was wrong with Deeno? What was the book about that he suggested Deeno should read?

- How did Deeno's life change with the book?

- What could the book help you with?

WHAT TO DO AND HOW TO DO IT!

Tensing and relaxing

First of all, I will be talking about the idea of *physical relaxation*.

When we are thinking of our body, relaxing means the opposite of tensing. The following exercise will show you what I am talking about:

- Make a strong fist with both hands. You are doing it right when you are feeling your nails digging into the palm of your hands and you see the knuckles of the outside of your hands almost going white.

- This is an example of creating tension.

- When you open up your fists, you release the tension and relax your hands. Experience how nice that feels.

- You can also do this with the muscles in your face.

- Open your eyes as wide as you can, wider, that's good, hold it.

- Now open your mouth as wide as you can, hold it, hold it, count quietly to five and release. Now feel the relaxation of your facial muscles. That feels very good, doesn't it?

Both of these exercises are examples of creating first physical *tension* and then physical *relaxation*, which feels very calming because certain muscles in your body go into holiday mode when you relax them. In the beginning, in order to get your whole body in this pleasant holiday mode, it is best if you do your relaxation exercises while lying down. Your body is automatically more comfortable using less of your muscles than when you are standing.

Second, when you are doing relaxation you should also try to *relax your thoughts*. I am sure you have heard your parents or other adults talk about wanting to relax. That means they want to be undisturbed for a while to get some peace and quiet. As I said before, relaxing is getting lots of rest just like on holiday after a long term at school. You don't want to think about your schoolwork or what you have to do next. You need stillness around you. No more talking, giggling or looking around.

Exercise: Close your eyes. Imagine that a big blue bubble slowly comes your way. It is beautiful. Just the colour and size you want it to be. When it is quite close, you take a step forward and enter the bubble. It immediately surrounds you like a protective, warm shield. You don't hear anything apart from your own breathing. It is so peaceful. Nobody can disturb you any more. You are safe and protected, feeling very calm and relaxed. Then, slowly count down from five to zero, open your eyes wide and have a good stretch.

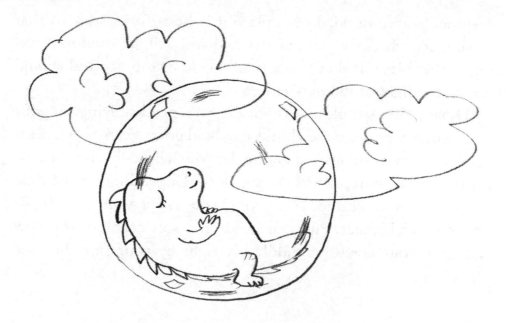

Points for discussion
• Can you see or visualize the bubble? How would you describe it to someone else?
• How does it feel to be in the bubble?
• What is physical relaxation?
• What is a way to relax your head?
• How do you feel now, after having done these exercises?

Finding and preparing a place for relaxation

It is very important that you find yourself a quiet place where you can get comfortable and do your relaxation. You want stillness around you to really be able to get into the exercises.

Once you've decided on a place it is best if you stick to that same place whenever you practise and you will get used to relaxing in that place. It should not be too cold or too hot and should not be too light or too dark either.

During the day, please do not do your practise lying on your bed, otherwise your mind thinks it should go to sleep. Get a blanket and a few cushions out and make yourself really comfortable for your relaxation practice on the floor. Depending on the time of the year and weather conditions, you might want to snuggle under a soft blanket. Put your head on a soft cushion or pillow and have your favourite cuddly toy right by your side. Just see

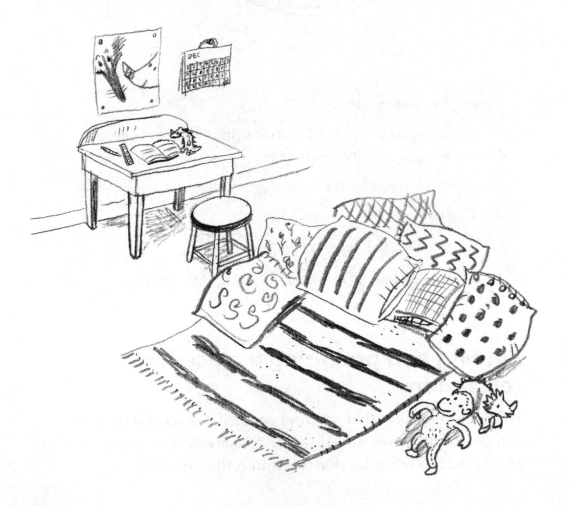

what is the best way for you to feel most comfortable on the floor. When practising relaxation it does not really matter what you are wearing except that it should be comfortable.

Tell your family, brothers and sisters to excuse you for a while. Then turn off any electrical equipment in the room that might distract you: mobile phone, radio/TV, stereo, computer. Close the door and the window if it is not too hot and sticky in that place to keep noise distraction to a minimum. I think it might be a great idea to get a sign 'No entry or do not disturb for a little while please, I am doing relaxation!' You can draw or paint it by hand or prepare one on the computer and print if off. You choose any method you like and you can be as creative as you want. Deeno also has a sign for his door:

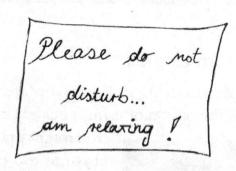

The practice postures
Lying down

This is most suitable for beginners. Your head is resting on a pillow, your arms are lying on either side of the body with your palms facing down and your feet are flopping to either side. Nothing is tight. You are relaxing all your muscles. They are on holiday mode. Now close your eyes: think of the big blue bubble that embraces you and slowly takes you up in the air...you are feeling very safe and protected...

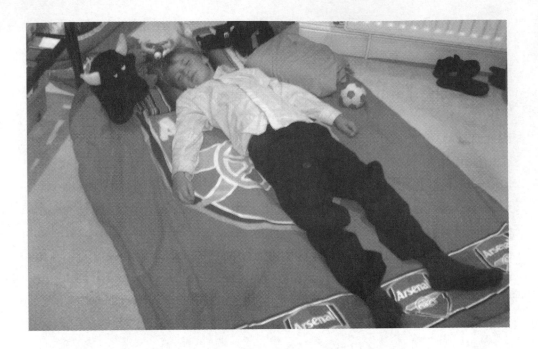

Sitting on a normal chair

If you cannot practise lying down or you are getting more advanced you have the option of using a chair. I could imagine that

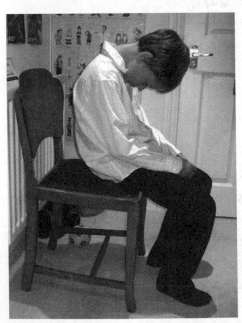

you might practise on the bus if it is not too busy or you might find a few minutes of peace and quiet on the toilet before a test or oral examination.

Sit on the front half of the chair with your feet shoulder width apart resting firmly on the floor. Your spine is first straight and then slumps and you gently bend over to the front with your head leaning forwards, resting your chin on your upper chest. Make sure your neck feels soft and keep your hands flat on each leg or folded in your lap. You are relaxing all your muscles. They are into holiday mode. Now close your eyes, think of a big blue bubble…it is your bubble…you are feeling very safe and protected…it is beautiful…

Body check

Once you've positioned yourself, do a quick all round body check to make sure you are really feeling comfortable and nothing feels tight or is distracting you, for example a belt or your glasses which you might want to take off for this exercise.

What happens each week in the programme

Step by step, I will tell you now exactly how your weekly relaxation sessions will work.

- Each week, together with your parent or another adult, you'll learn new magic words and the changes in your body you need to concentrate on. Learn the name of the new magic words according to where you are in the programme. Read the magic words in the cloud several times out loud to become very familiar with them.

- Understand what the magic words are doing to your body and actively imagine feeling this. This is called visualization and is very powerful!

- Look at the activities that go with the magic words. They will help you to get into the right mood. If you have enough time, choose one that you want to do.

- Lie on your blanket, read the story that goes with the magic words, or get someone to read the story of the week to you, whilst quietly repeating the magic words in your mind as you hear the magic words mentioned in the story. Concentrate on actively imagining you are feeling the changes in your body taking place.

- After the story, there is always a little explanation to help you with your own practice during the week.

- Finally, do the suggested follow-up activity to get the most out of learning the new magic words – unless, of course, it is bedtime and you are ready to go to sleep.

In this relaxation technique, you have to repeat all magic words roughly three to six times quietly in your head. There is no need to count very seriously. What is important is that you are feeling the change in your body that you are meant to create with concentrating on the magic words. It will all become very clear to you once you've started.

During the six weeks, you will find that every day is different and you may not be equally successful each day with your practice. Some exercises will have an immediate effect whereas with others it will take longer for you to feel the desired result. That is absolutely normal. We all have good and bad days and this will be reflected in your daily practice. When you are feeling tense after a stressful day, it will be more challenging to relax into the exercises. That is to be expected. You didn't learn to read over night, did you? All learning takes time. Just do it! Daily! There will be results!

Closing the exercises

Unless you are doing the exercises in bed before sleeping, it is important to come to a proper end after the exercise(s). It's just like when you go cycling. Imagine a bicycle in front of you. Before you start riding it, it is important for you to know how to stop again, isn't it? It is the same with this relaxation technique. To 'close' the exercise means we are coming out of the holiday mode, we are leaving the blue bubble:

- Make a strong fist with both hands.

- Bend/flex your elbows sharply several times.

- Open your eyes wide.

- Take a few deep breaths and have a good stretch.

- You are now feeling wide awake and energetic.

Exception

As I mentioned above, please do not close the exercise when you are practising in bed at night. At this time of the day, the exercise is designed to help you to fall asleep more quickly. Just do the exercise as usual and then take the pleasant feelings of relaxation and calmness with you into your sleep. You will have lovely dreams.

Setting up a routine
Practice makes perfect!

Just like learning any new skill it is important to do it regularly. Remember when you started to ride your bike: it was quite a challenge, wasn't it? After doing it again and again, maybe having had a little fall here and there, it started to become easier and even fun. It gave you a real feeling of pride the first time you rode your bike without any help and without falling off. This is the same with this relaxation technique. The good thing is practice is short:

- Do three minutes in the morning before going to school.

- Do three minutes after coming back from school, before doing anything else.

- Do three minutes at night before falling asleep when lying in bed.

Make it part of your daily routine just like brushing your teeth and washing your hands when you get back from school. If you do it regularly you will quickly feel the change in you.

To practise on your own:

1. Find a quiet place to sit or lie down.

2. Close your eyes and think of the bubble coming your way, taking you to an imaginary far away place.

3. Say the magic words quietly in your head.

4. Concentrate on feeling the changes in your body.

5. Don't forget to close the exercise at the end unless it is bedtime.

6. Feel calm and refreshed!

What the relaxation technique can help you with

- Being able to go on a little holiday in your mind no matter where you are (even if you are at home).

- Feeling really energized after a few minutes of practice and getting your homework done in no time.

- Calming down before a test or when having to go to the doctor or anywhere that makes you feel anxious.

- Falling asleep more quickly and feeling more rested when waking up.

- Staying happy and healthy.

- No longer being afraid in the dark or of being alone.

- Not getting a headache any more.

- Healing allergies or skin problems.

- Liking and loving yourself more.

- Being courageous and feeling strong.

I reckon that's worth practising regularly, don't you?

How to use the practice plan

On the next page you can see the practice plan. You can either write in the book or photocopy it and keep it somewhere safe.

Try and fill it in on a daily basis; perhaps in the evening before going to bed. Every box for each day is divided into three slots, one for the morning, one for the afternoon and one for the evening:

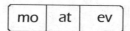

When you do your practice, put a smiley face in the right box. It does not matter when you do it; however, establish a routine and always do it at the same time. That way, your body clock will get programmed and will remind you when it's time to relax for a few minutes.

At the end of each week, maybe on Sunday evenings, add up the number of smiley faces and write the number underneath each week. The more smiley faces, the more relaxed you will feel.

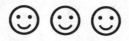

Relaxation diary for 6 weeks

Draw ☹ or ☺ into the boxes [ ][ ][ ]   ☺ if you practised   ☹ if you didn't practise

	Week 1	Week 2	Week 3	Week 4	Week 5	Week 6
Date:						
Mon						
Tue						
Wed						
Thu						
Fri						
Sat						
Sun						
How many times did you practise?						

☺ ☺ ☺ ☺ ☺ ...

Tips and reminders

1. When you are first starting out with the six week programme, it is best to practise lying down. Your body knows this position from when you go to sleep and will relax more quickly than in a seated position.

2. Practise at least three times daily, keep it short but regular. You will soon feel the benefits.

3. Always practise in the same place and at the same time so your body can get used to it. Make it a daily ritual like brushing your teeth.

4. Part of a ritual can also be objects, the same objects each time which you have chosen to make part of your routine; i.e. the same soft cushions, a soft toy, maybe a scented candle or an incense/oil burner with a few drops of calming lavender or vanilla oil, a yoga mat or a blanket; anything to get you really cosy.

5. It is absolutely vital that it is very quiet around you. All electrical items, i.e. TV, stereo, iPod, mobile phone, etc., need to be temporarily switched off so you can really get into your private 'holiday mode' for a little while.

6. In order to remind your family that you are practising put up a 'Please do not disturb' sign on the door of the room where you are practising.

7. Food or drink must not be part of the practice because it only distracts you and would stop your mind from concentrating on the magic words.

8. Should you find it hard to get into the practice it might be an idea to imagine pictures. Perhaps pictures of little

Deeno, the dinosaur who accompanies you through this book and all the exercises. You could also draw your own picture before the exercise and concentrate on it later during the exercise when saying the magic words. This process of imagining your own pictures is called visualization and can be very powerful.

9. Most important of all is that you have an enormous amount of patience with yourself. You cannot learn the exercises overnight. There will be days when it does not work according to plan and that is normal. The next day it will be easier again.

10. The same applies to the magic words. Make sure you know how to apply the magic words really well and notice the changes in your body before starting to set up and use your own magic words.

With regular practice, you will soon become much calmer, stronger and truly confident. Good luck!

Part C

The Six-Week Programme

THE RELAXATION PROGRAMME

WEEK 1: 'CALMNESS, HEAVINESS'

The purpose of the calmness magic words is to get you into the mood for relaxation. These are the magic words you will always start out with, whatever week of the programme you are on.

The calmness magic words are…

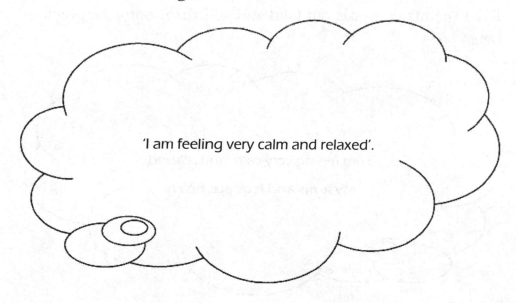

'I am feeling very calm and relaxed'.

Say these words three times to tune into the relaxation exercises in your head and with your body. Try and imagine a big bubble coming your way, that you enter, and that will surround you with perfect peacefulness and quiet. You will hear more about the bubble soon.

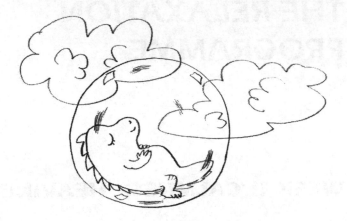

Continue with heaviness.

The heaviness magic words are...

'My arms and legs are heavy'.

Read the magic words out loud and add them onto the previous ones

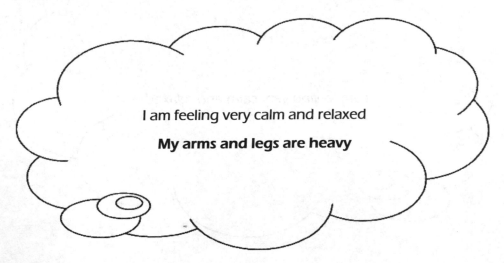

What happens? With this exercise your muscles will start to relax. First you'll feel it in your arms and legs and then everywhere in your body.

What's the purpose? When the muscles in your body start to loosen up and relax, it gets easier for the blood to flow around more evenly. This is what makes your body feel heavy and generally more and more relaxed.

Points for discussion

When have you felt heavy in your arms and legs before?

- Maybe when carrying a shopping bag, or your school bag?

- Or perhaps after running around a lot and when playing sports?

- Or how about going up a steep flight of stairs?

Next time you are doing this, watch yourself and feel that feeling of heaviness in your legs. Whatever you remember, it must be a positive memory otherwise you won't be able to relax. You can visualize any of the above-mentioned scenarios to help you with your own relaxation practice during the rest of the week.

WARM-UP ACTIVITY

✏ **No equipment needed but possibly a bit of space to move around – you could play some uplifting music to make it more fun but it is not necessary.**

Imagine you are a heavy animal; maybe an elephant or a hippo. Just think about what your chosen animal looks like. In your mind, you observe how it moves. What do the legs do…, the head… and the rest of the body? Is it very light or rather heavy in its movements? Does it take big or small steps? Its muscles are very heavy and so are its arms and legs. Imagine how it feels to have such heavy limbs. Now try to move exactly like that animal. Walk around a little bit just like that animal would move. Remember how heavy its legs are and its head as well. Once you've felt what it is like to have such heavy arms and legs lie down on the floor like this heavy animal. Really visualize this heavy animal and feel it in your own body.

You can now start the heaviness exercise, saying the two sets of magic words 'I am feeling calm and relaxed' plus the new heaviness magic words, quietly in your mind. Read the story yourself or listen to it being read to you. Lie down/sit down and simply be aware of whether the changes in your body that you want to create are taking place. Can you feel the heaviness in your limbs? Don't forget to 'close' the exercise properly at the end unless this is bedtime for you (see 'Closing the exercises', p.58).

THE HEAVINESS STORY

The Friendly, Furry Creatures

You are lying on a soft blanket on the floor and you are starting to become relaxed. You are taking a deep breath in mhh…and then an even longer breath out phooooo… That's it. Really good. You are taking another big breath in, you are breathing in gentleness and softness and breathing out all the bad things…you are letting go of all of them… Excellent. As you are concentrating on your breathing you don't even notice that a big, blue bubble has slowly come your way. It is beautiful. Before you know it, it surrounds you like a protective, warm shield. You don't hear anything apart from your own breathing. It is so peaceful. Nobody can disturb you any more. You are safe and protected. You lie down, close your eyes and *you are feeling very calm and relaxed*. Everything seems really, really far away and you are getting very comfortable in the bubble as you are setting off on your journey.

After a while, you wake up and you see that you are surrounded by lots of smiling, furry creatures. You start laughing. 'Where am I?' One really big, heavy creature comes forward; he almost seems a bit shy: 'Hello, you wonderful little person,' he says. 'Welcome to Heavy-land. It's great to have you here. Will you come and play with us? Everybody here is very heavy and very friendly.' You have a quick look around and you see a huge field with red poppies, bright blue cornflowers and big yellow sunflowers with long pretty leaves. You become aware of the fantastic scent these flowers give out. It smells wonderful. You play with the heavy, furry, smiley creatures, and they keep on saying: *1, 2, 3, 4, 5 – mine is a happy life! 1, 2, 3, 4, 5 – mine is a happy life! 1, 2, 3, 4, 5 – mine is a happy life!* And you join in…you are feeling so happy. They all want to be next to you, hold your hand and smile at you. You are playing hide and seek in the field and behind the trees, you are running around, chasing a colourful butterfly and you try to walk like the heavy, furry, friendly creatures.

You observe their heavy steps and the gentle rocking from one side to the other, from left to right and right to left and again left to right as they move forward. It creates a fun little rhythmic movement. You all end up walking in a big circle, in heavy, slow steps, one after the other, rocking from left to right and right to left and you all start singing in a low, deep voice: *My arms and legs feel really heavy. My arms and legs feel really heavy. My arms and legs feel really heavy.* And you can feel there is a real heaviness in your arms. Your legs are feeling equally heavy, so heavy. You are feeling very heavy all over and you are lying down on the floor like all the heavy, furry, friendly creatures. You notice the beautiful smell in the air, and you can hear the wind as it is playing with the flowers in the field and the leaves of the trees. You like that rustling sound, it is very soothing. Eventually, you feel your body filling up with

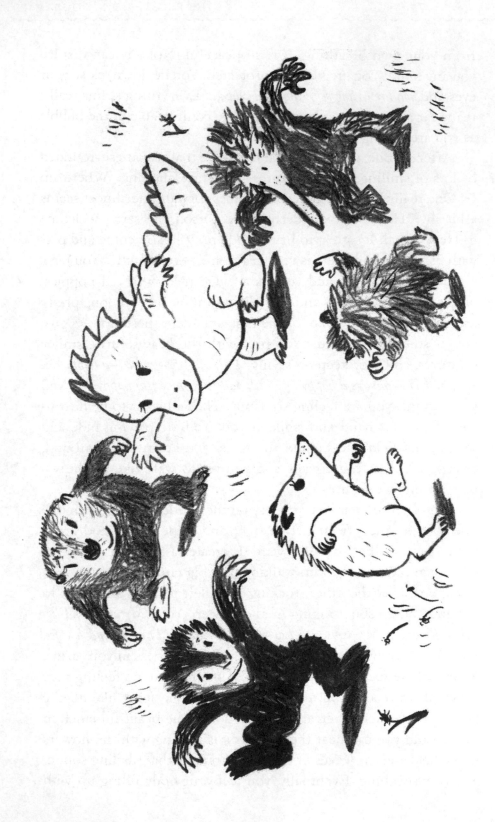

new energy. You are feeling strong. You get up, say good-bye to the heavy, furry, friendly creatures, wave to the butterfly and the big blue bubble takes you back home. It is only now that you realize that you are clenching something in your fist. As you open your hand you find a little, furry, heavy stone. You are so happy because you know that holding this stone can take you back any time to the heavy, friendly, furry creatures, where you can do anything you like and feel energized, happy and strong. Just imagine that big blue bubble around you, hold onto the stone and there you are in the field. This is your place. No-one else knows how to get to it but you. You are returning home, very happy and full of energy.

Now get ready to leave the big blue bubble…'close' the exercise, and come out of the holiday mode:

- Make a strong fist with both hands.

- Bend/flex your elbows sharply several times.

- Open your eyes wide.

- Take a few deep breaths and have a good stretch.

ON YOUR OWN THIS WEEK

This is what you do to practise the heaviness magic words during the week.

1. Find a quiet place to sit or lie down.

2. Close your eyes and think of the bubble coming your way, taking you to an imaginary far away place with wonderfully friendly heavy creatures.

3. Repeat three to six times quietly in your head:

> **I am feeling very calm and relaxed**
>
> **My arms and legs are heavy**

4. Concentrate on feeling the heaviness in your arms and legs as if you had just been running around in the playground or walked up a steep flight of stairs.

5. Don't forget to close the exercise at the end unless it is bedtime.

FOLLOW-UP ACTIVITIES

✏ **You will need: either just paper and colouring pens or also old newspaper/magazines, a pair of scissors, sticky tape and some cardboard, elastic bands/a piece of string.**

1. Take some paper, colouring pens, crayons or watercolour paints and a paint brush and draw or paint that heavy animal exactly how you imagined it.

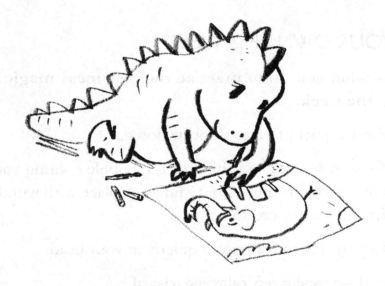

2. Take some old newspaper or magazines and a pair of scissors and cut the animal shape out of the newspaper, stick it onto cardboard and colour it in. I am sure you can think of more heavy animals and, if you like, you can make them as well.

3. Draw a face mask to represent that heavy animal. Don't forget to cut in holes for the nose and mouth, attach a piece of string on each side, put it over your face and then dance and move around like this animal again. If you want, you can play music to accompany your little dance. Whatever you choose to do, it will help you to learn the heaviness exercise.

WEEK 2: 'WARMTH'

The warmth magic words are…

'My arms and legs are warm'.

Read the magic words out loud and add them on to the previous magic words.

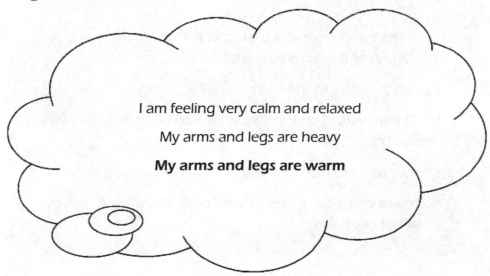

I am feeling very calm and relaxed

My arms and legs are heavy

My arms and legs are warm

What happens? Your muscles will be relaxing with this exercise so that your blood is flowing like wonderful, hot chocolate sauce through your body making you feel nice and warm all over.

What's the purpose? If you are really concentrating very hard on feeling warmth in your body, really imagining how your whole body is slowly warming up starting with your arms and legs, your blood vessels will relax. They will get bigger and this means that more blood can flow into your skin. Maybe, you will be feeling a slight tingling sensation in your feet and/or hands. If you often have cold hands or feet, this exercise could change that after a few weeks of regular practice.

Points for discussion

When have you felt pleasantly warm before? What memories do you hold of feeling lovely and warm?

- In winter time: you are sitting in a cosy room in front of the warm fire place.

- Maybe when coming home after playing outdoors on a cold day and your hands and feet are slowly warming up?

- In the summer: you are lying in the grass, the sun is shining and warms your body.

- You are lying in the bath.

- You are sitting on the sofa wrapped up in a cuddly warm blanket.

- Your feet are nice and warm in lovely woollen socks.

- You've come back from a long walk, drinking a nice cup of hot chocolate.

This is exactly the feeling you want to create with this exercise. Everyone has different memories. Make sure yours is a very positive one and it will certainly help you with these magic words.

WARM-UP ACTIVITIES

✏ **No equipment needed but a bit of space for child(ren) to move around – some music can be played but it is not necessary.**

1. Put your hands under running warm water for a while. It is a good way to experience the difference in how your hands feel before, during and after the warm water has warmed them up. This may help you to imagine an increased sense of warmth in your body.

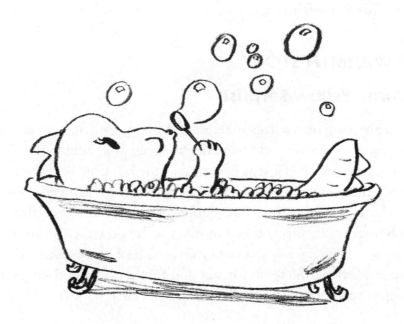

2. As you can see in the picture, Deeno is having a lovely bath and is really enjoying it.

At home:
How about getting some exciting blue bubble bath and doing the same in preparation for the exercise? You can also have a shower; obviously, you cannot blow bubbles but it has a similar effect in terms of making you feel nice and warm inside and out.

When not at home:
Draw yourself or Deeno in the bath at home, or describe what it feels like to be in the bath or shower and the changes in your body/skin temperature afterwards. Close your eyes and recall that comfortable feeling after a bath or hot shower.

With that comforting feeling of warmth you can now start the warmth exercise, saying all the magic words quietly in your mind or listening to the story being read to you. Lie down/sit down and simply be aware of whether the changes in your body that you want to create are taking place. Can you feel the warmth in your limbs? Don't forget to 'close' the exercise properly at the end unless this is bedtime for you.

THE WARMTH STORY

A Warm, Yellow Surprise

You are lying on a soft blanket on the floor again and *you are feeling very calm and relaxed* and you notice that big blue bubble has slowly come your way. It is just as beautiful as the last time you saw it. You really like how it feels to be surrounded by its protective, warm shield. It is so peaceful in the bubble. This is your secret place and nobody can disturb you any more. You lie down, close your eyes and *you are feeling very calm and relaxed*. The bubble takes off into the air, leaving the town further and further behind disappearing deeper and deeper into the blue sky. [PAUSE]

After a while you wake up and you see a big yellow sunray shining into the bubble. This looks very inviting, you think. You hop up and start carefully climbing up the sunray that looks a bit like a strong yellow ribbon coming down from the sun. It is holding you very safely and you become more courageous and climb higher and higher towards the sun. Around you is nothing but the clear blue sky. You have been climbing the sunray for quite some time when you start feeling a little tired and you decide to take a break. You get comfortable on the sunray and realize how heavy your arms and legs are feeling from all this tough climbing. *Your arms and legs are feeling really heavy* and suddenly you are thinking how peaceful it is up here, high above the towns, country lanes, fields, rivers and far away from everybody else. You get a feeling of deep satisfaction

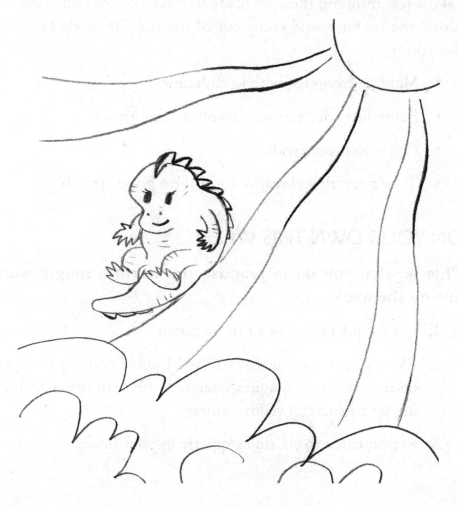

and gratefulness inside, you are so happy to have found this place. You take in the comforting warmth of the sunray underneath you. *Your arms and legs feel really warm.* The sunray is sending you pleasant warmth and your body feels nice and warm all over. It is a very nurturing sunray giving you lots of new energy and strength. Take in as much as you want. Take your time…

[PAUSE]

…and when you are really energized and your fuel tank is filled up you will sit up on the sunray, take a few deep breaths and slide back down into the bubble. Weeeeee…sliding down is so much fun and you are going quite fast…back down into the bubble, which is now bringing you safely back into this room.

Take a few minutes, then get ready to leave the big blue bubble… 'close' the exercise, and come out of the holiday mode back into this room:

- Make a strong fist with both hands.

- Bend/flex your elbows sharply several times.

- Open your eyes wide.

- Take a few deep breaths and have a good stretch.

ON YOUR OWN THIS WEEK

This is what you do to practise the warmth magic words during the week.

1. Find a quiet place to sit or lie down.

2. Close your eyes and think of the bubble coming your way, taking you to an imaginary far away place in the sky, climbing up a beautiful yellow sunray.

3. Repeat three to six times quietly in your head:

I am feeling very calm and relaxed

My arms and legs are heavy

My arms and legs are warm

4. Concentrate on feeling the warmth in your arms and legs, remembering the pleasantly warm sunray.

5. Don't forget to close the exercise at the end unless it is bedtime.

FOLLOW-UP ACTIVITIES

You can choose to do both or just one of the suggestions. This will help you to remember the magic words.

> ✏ **You will need:**
> **Paper, colouring pens/crayons/watercolour paints.**

1. Take some paper and choose whatever you prefer; colouring pens, crayons or watercolour paints and a paint brush. Remember, as I explained earlier, how these magic words will help your muscles to relax so that your blood is flowing like wonderful, hot chocolate sauce evenly through your body making you feel nice and warm all over.

   Now, I would like you to draw or paint how Deeno is lying in bed, very relaxed, as the yummy chocolate sauce is gliding around in his body, warming up every single part of him. Make sure you give him a big smile on his face. Remember, he is feeling great after that blue bubble bath and I hope you are very calm and happy too, after just having done the 'Warmth' exercise.

2. Think about colours in general. There are so many, but which colour do you feel is a cold colour and which one is a warm colour? Once you have decided, I would like you to make a picture using only 'warm' colours and think about situations in which you first felt really cold and then warm. For example, coming inside after having played outdoors on a winter's day and sitting by the fire, having a bath, holding your favourite cuddly toy, etc. I am sure you can think of many more.

Next time, when you are having a bath or a shower, try to be really aware of how that warmth feels inside and how your skin feels afterwards when you are lying in bed.

WEEK 3: 'BREATHING'

The breathing magic words are…

'My breathing is calm and regular'.

Read the new magic words out loud, then add them to last week's words.

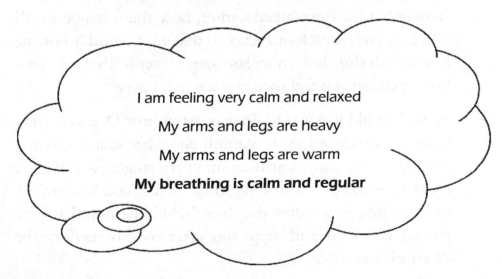

I am feeling very calm and relaxed

My arms and legs are heavy

My arms and legs are warm

My breathing is calm and regular

What happens? In this exercise you are observing how your breath is very regular without you having to do anything actively. When we feel calm, breathing in and out is like the regular rhythm of an old clock's pendulum.

What's the purpose? In this exercise we are trying to develop greater awareness of the calm rhythm of our breathing and where our breath is going in the body. We are quietly observing our breathing and it is very calming to feel and become more aware of the regular rhythm of the chest moving up and down. It is just like the wind that creates waves when playing with the water. If you are really concentrating very hard on simply observing, not doing anything, nothing can interfere and you are feeling very, very calm. After a few weeks of practising these magic words, you will notice that even in tricky situations when you start to feel nervous your breathing will be calm if you quietly say the magic words in your head.

Points for discussion

- What do we need to survive?

- How long can we live without food? How often do you think about food and eating?

- How long can we live without water? How often do you think about drinking?

- How long can we live without breathing? What does that tell you about the importance of breathing? Yet, how often do you think about breathing?

Survival depends on many factors; one can actually survive for much longer without food than without water. In very hot conditions people cannot go without water for more than two days.

Some people can go without food for one or two months whereas others can only survive for one week.

However, breathing correctly is what keeps us alive. It normally happens automatically. Just occasionally, when you are very nervous or anxious or after having been running in the playground, you can be out of breath. This means your body has to breathe harder and faster than normal to supply your body with more oxygen.

This week's magic words will help you to keep your breathing calm and healthy. It helps you to get in tune with a slow, regular rhythmic movement, like your stomach going gently up and down as you are breathing in and out.

WARM-UP ACTIVITIES

> ✏ **You will need: balloons to blow up, a bit of space to run on the spot – possibly accompanied by some music.**

1. Experimenting with your breath.

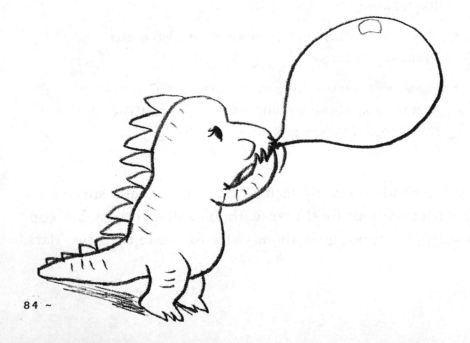

First of all I'd like you to place your hands on the left and right hand side of your rib cage just underneath your chest; that's it. Now take a deep breath in, hold it and feel how your ribs open up under your hands. Now let go of your breath and feel how the rib cage goes small again and sinks down as you are breathing out. Underneath your rib cage are your lungs which can blow up like a balloon. Have you ever seen what happens to a balloon if you let go of it? Exactly, it goes all thin and loses all the air. The same happens to your lungs as you breathe out.

2. Working with a balloon.

If you happen to have a balloon, I'd like you to blow it up right now and I want you to observe what happens in your body. Where does the air you are blowing into the balloon come from? Where does it go to? Can you influence the air? How about holding your breath for a short moment and then blow out really carefully and slowly. Can you play with the rhythm of the air? Try it, if you can; what is it like to take the air from deep down out of your stomach? What is it like getting the air for the balloon out of your chest area?

3. Snake-breathing.

Imagine you are a big snake. The snake takes a deep breath through its nose into its tummy. Keep it there for a moment. Now put your teeth together and as you are opening your lips, you start breathing out, taking your time, making a loud 'sssssssss' sound just like snakes do. Repeat this five times. In the snake language it means: 'I want to be left alone. I do not want anybody to distract me!'

4. Running on the spot.

Another possibility for you to experience your breath is to run on the spot. Start fairly slowly and then go faster and faster and faster... Go, go go. What happens? You are getting out of breath? That's good. Your body is breathing much faster now because it needs more oxygen.

Having experienced your breathing in this way, you can now start the *breathing exercise*: say all the magic words, including the new breathing magic words, quietly in your mind or listen to the story being read to you. Lie down/sit down and simply be aware of whether the changes in your body that you want to create are taking place. Be the silent observer of your breathing. Can you feel the rhythmic up and down of your chest? It is all happening without you having to do anything. Don't forget to 'close' the exercise properly at the end unless this is bedtime for you.

THE BREATHING STORY

The Rainbow Run

You are lying on a soft blanket on the floor and you are starting to feel relaxed. You are taking a deep breath in mhh...and then an even longer breath out phooooo... That's it. Really good. You had a tough day today and you are feeling exhausted, not wanting to do anything but relax for a while... No sooner have you had these ideas than the big blue bubble arrives and picks you up to take you far away to a magic place. Oh, how you love being in that bubble. It is so cosy and comfortable and it always knows new places to take you to...

You are drifting in the air, floating over houses, villages, fields, trees... and *you are feeling very calm and relaxed*. You are thinking about a place that you will be taken to...and suddenly you see yourself running...you are running towards Deeno who is standing at the other end of a colourful...well, what is it? You can't really see it... It looks like a long, soft ribbon...it is making a big curve and you have to run upwards but it is as if magic feet were carrying you. You are as fast as the wind and before you know it Deeno is putting his short little arms around you to give you a big hug. That feels so good. Deeno has become such a great friend. Now, looking up, you realize that you are standing in the middle, right at the very top, of a beautiful, big rainbow.

All those gorgeous colours… You have just been running over a rainbow…and with that thought you lie down on the soft rainbow floor and you begin to feel your heavy arms and legs from all that running…*your arms and legs feel really heavy* and the sun is shining

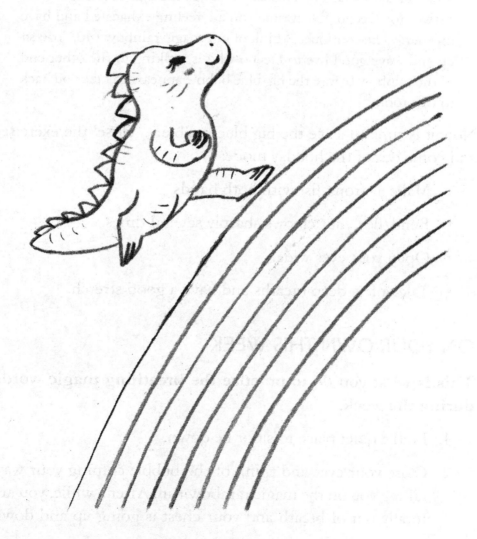

down on you from above, sending you warmth and happiness… *your arms and legs feel really warm.* You are feeling warm and relaxed all over. The wind is picking up slightly and the rainbow gently rocks from side to side…taking you deeper and deeper into a comforting state of soft relaxation. Your breathing has slowed down and you notice that the up and down in your chest is becoming a very slow, steady movement. *Your breathing is calm and regular.* It is breathing inside you…there is nothing you need to do…[PAUSE]…then you hear a gentle whisper: 'Hey you, it's time to go back.' It is Deeno, whispering into your ear. 'Did you have a nice time on the rainbow?' he asks you. The relaxed smile in your eyes is enough of an answer for Deeno. 'Next time you are feeling exhausted and have no energy,' he continues, 'think of our magic rainbow run.' You sit up and wave good-bye to Deeno who is walking to the other end of the rainbow before the big blue bubble appears to take you back to this room.

Now it is time to leave the big blue bubble… 'close' the exercise, and come out of the holiday mode:

- Make a strong fist with both hands.

- Bend/flex your elbows sharply several times.

- Open your eyes wide.

- Take a few deep breaths and have a good stretch.

ON YOUR OWN THIS WEEK

This is what you do to practise the breathing magic words during the week.

1. Find a quiet place to sit or lie down.

2. Close your eyes and think of the bubble coming your way, taking you on the magic rainbow run. After a while, you are totally out of breath and your chest is going up and down

with heavy breathing. As you are resting on the rainbow, the wind starts to pick up, rocking you and the rainbow very gently from side to side. Your chest movements are beginning to slow down, you are starting to feel very calm. It is very soothing to feel your own breathing taking on a very regular rhythmic movement. It has a calming effect on you.

3. Say quietly in your head:

> I am feeling very calm and relaxed
>
> My arms and legs are heavy
>
> My arms and legs are warm
>
> **My breathing is calm and regular**

4. Concentrate on feeling the regular heartbeat in your body and remembering the rainbow's soothing, rhythmic rocking while resting on it after your run.

5. Don't forget to close the exercise at the end unless it is bedtime.

FOLLOW-UP ACTIVITIES

✏ **You will need:**

1. **paper, colouring pens/crayons/water paints**
2. **straws, peas and two plates between two children.**

1. If you feel like it, you can take some paper and work with colouring pens, crayons or watercolour paints and a paint brush. I would like you to remember situations where your

breathing stopped for a second because you were so excited and happy that you forgot to breathe. Maybe you've been to the circus before and have seen the acrobats high above you doing some amazing stunts. It certainly takes your breath away watching a tightrope artist walking from one end of the rope to the other, balancing the body extremely skilfully. You can certainly hear a pin drop when all the faces in the audience are captivated, drawn towards the one point high above in the big circus tent. How about drawing little Deeno as a tightrope walker?

2. Alternatively, you can pretend to be on a swing or a tree in the wind or a boat being rocked slowly from side to side on the water. This is to show how your breath moves in a wonderful rhythm, especially after having done this exercise for a while. How about drawing a young tree blowing in the wind, or Deeno in a boat or on a swing?

3. It is also good fun to discover your breath with a straw. Get a few peas from the kitchen, put them onto one plate and have an empty one a little further away from you on the floor. Now use your breath and the straw to transport the peas one at a time from one plate to the other. In this game, it is great to compete with your brother or sister or a friend.

WEEK 4: 'HEART'

The heart magic words are...

'My heartbeat is calm and regular'.

Read the new magic words before you add this one onto the previous ones.

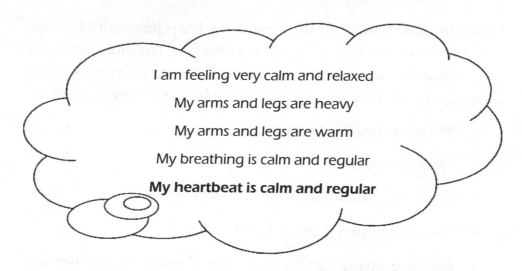

I am feeling very calm and relaxed

My arms and legs are heavy

My arms and legs are warm

My breathing is calm and regular

My heartbeat is calm and regular

What happens? This exercise is about you feeling your heart or your pulse beating. You see, your heartbeat gets passed on in the form of the pulse into other areas and blood vessels of your body. The moment that you start to feel your own rhythmic heartbeat you are entering further into a deep and pleasant state of relaxation.

What's the purpose? This is supposed to make you aware of how very relaxing it is for you and your body when your heart is beating calmly and steadily.

Points for discussion

I am sure you can think of many occasions when you really felt your heart beating strongly. Have a think...

- when playing sports, on your birthday, opening presents or watching your friends coming to celebrate with you

- before and during any happy event in your life, for example, when you saw a little puppy dog waddling towards you, wagging its tail with excitement

- or when someone has said loving things to you.

I am sure you've heard of the phrase 'my heart leapt with joy'?!

Our heart is very sensitive when it comes to emotions; pleasant and unpleasant ones alike! This is why there are so many sayings about the heart. Can you think of any? Here are a few examples:

- 'My heart leapt with joy'

- 'My heart sank'

- 'This came from the bottom of my heart'

- ' I could not find it in my heart to say...'

- 'She is wearing her heart on her sleeve!' or, last but not least,

- 'He has a heart of gold'.

Put your hand onto your heart and feel how it's beating. At this stage, you might not be able to pick up a very strong heartbeat. It might be rather faint. What I want you to concentrate on with the heart magic words is getting better at feeling your heart or your pulse beating very happily and regularly.

WARM-UP ACTIVITIES

✏ **You will need: a bit of space to dance – possibly accompanied by some fun music**

1. Put the middle finger of your left hand on the inside of your right wrist and try to find your pulse.

2. Imagine you are holding a little kitten or a puppy dog sitting on your lap and you feel its heartbeat.

3. Now I would like you to put on some funky music and imagine it has started raining hearts, lots and lots of hearts, and you are running and dancing around, trying to catch as many as you can and put them into a secret basket.

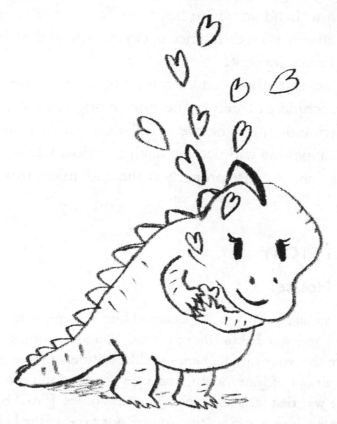

There are many more hearts; run and catch them all. Wonderful. Catch the ones high up and the ones just about to land on the floor. Catch the ones in the left top corner, the right top corner. Jump up to really reach the hearts and dance with your basket full of hearts… Can you start to feel your heart beating a little faster? Put your hand onto your heart and feel how it's beating now that you've been dancing around. I bet you can feel it much more now?! You see, there is so much life in you. Now sit down next to your secret basket. Take a few hearts from your basket in your hands, close your eyes and take the opportunity to send love out to children and people of your choice, to areas of conflict, to those in hospital, to those who are sad, who have lost a loved one and so on. You can always take more hearts out of your basket. There are plenty to give away...

Now, put your hand onto your heart and feel how it's beating – there should be a marked difference between now and before you did the heart dance exercise!

You can now start the heart exercise: say all the magic words quietly in your mind or listen to the story being read to you. Lie down/sit down and simply be the silent observer of your heart-beat. It is all happening without you having to do anything. Don't forget to 'close' the exercise properly at the end unless this is bed-time for you.

THE HEART STORY

The Secret House

There you are again in your big blue bubble. You are lying on a soft blanket and you are starting to relax. You are taking a deep breath in mhh…your tummy blows up like a little balloon. Then you let the air out of your mouth, making a gentle aahhh sound… you like the way that feels and repeat it several times. [PAUSE] All of a sudden you become aware that you are not alone in the bubble, there is someone else breathing just like you…who is this? It is Deeno. His face is beaming and he snuggles right up to you. 'I like this breathing, it relaxes me, *I am feeling very calm and relaxed*,' he says. And you too start *to feel very calm and relaxed, very calm and relaxed.*

You must have both dozed off for a while and when you open your eyes again you can hardly believe where the big blue bubble has taken you: you are deep down at the bottom of the sea, sur-rounded by water, and there are lots of colourful fish of all shapes and sizes who are staring at you with their big round smiley eyes. They are very friendly but also very curious about the two of you in that big blue bubble. You start to swim with them and you are surprised that you can breathe under water. It's as if a spell has come over you. Deeno is holding onto your hand and together you are feeling very safe swimming amongst the fish. It is a magic world under water, everything is so bright and there is so much to see…

It is wonderful. [PAUSE]

Suddenly, you come to an old house made of corals and shells. The door opens and a tiny shiny seahorse comes to welcome you and Deeno inside. You are swimming over a carpet of soft algae, which looks very inviting…you both feel like lying down. You realize how tired you are from the long swim and playing with the fish. Deeno is still holding your hand. You close your eyes and become

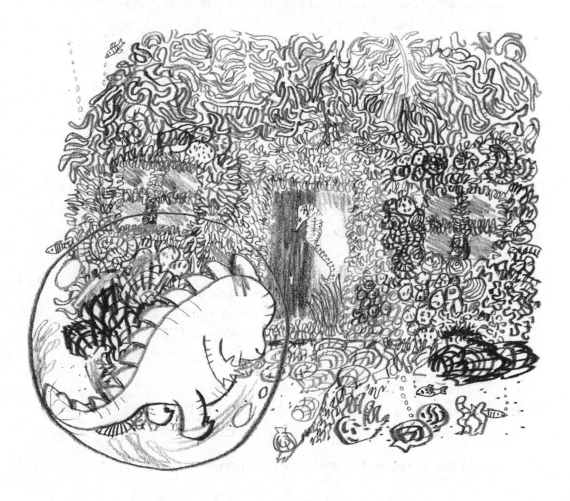

aware of your body being supported by this soft sea-carpet. *Your arms and legs feel really heavy* and they are also feeling really warm. *Your arms and legs feel really warm.* You are enjoying the quietness around you in this little house at the bottom of the sea. And when you notice the slow rhythmic up and down of Deeno's chest next to you which is very soothing *your own breathing is also becoming very calm and regular.*

[PAUSE]

A little red fish followed you into the house. You feel the little bubbles he is producing as they gently brush your face and notice their soft gargling sound as they pass by your ears. It has a very calming effect on you and your heart…*your heartbeat is now very calm and regular.* You are feeling so deeply relaxed as you are lying there on the soft carpet of the coral house and *you know: to be at rest is best! To be at rest is best!* [PAUSE]

Then you become aware of somebody standing by your side. You open your eyes and notice the tiny, shiny, seahorse: 'It is time to go,' it says, 'your bubble is waiting outside!' You wake Deeno up and together you swim out of the coral house and into the bubble. As it is slowly taking you away from the sea bottom you wave good-bye to the friendly seahorse, all the fish and you smile at Deeno: 'I had a wonderful time, didn't you?' He nods, still amazed by the vastness and magic beauty of the sea-world.

Very happy and full of energy you are returning home and you know that in your own mind you can always return to this special place whenever you need to feel calm and relaxed. This can be in the morning before going to school, at break time at school and at home. You can just close your eyes for a few minutes, imagine the bubble, Deeno and the beautiful sea world, quietly say your magic words and notice how good that makes you feel. The more often you say the magic words quietly in your mind, the more calm and relaxed you will feel in any situation.

In a few minutes, I would like you to get ready to 'close' the exercise, and come out of the sea-world mode:

- Make a strong fist with both hands.

- Bend/flex your elbows sharply several times.

- Open your eyes wide.

- Take a few deep breaths and have a good stretch.

ON YOUR OWN THIS WEEK

This is what you do to practise the heart magic words during the week.

1. Find a quiet place to sit or lie down.

2. Close your eyes and think of the bubble coming your way, taking you to an imaginary far away place in the sea with a coral house and amazing colours and shapes of fish and other water creatures. Feel how their gentle gargling sounds, the warm water and the gentle swimming have a very calming effect on your heartbeat.

3. Repeat three to six times quietly in your head:

   I am feeling very calm and relaxed

   My arms and legs are heavy

   My arms and legs are warm

   My breathing is calm and regular

   My heartbeat is calm and regular

4. Concentrate on feeling the regular heartbeat in your body as if listening to the ticking of a big old clock or maybe remembering the feeling of a little kitten's heartbeat as you are holding it in your arms.

5. Don't forget to close the exercise at the end unless it is bedtime.

FOLLOW-UP ACTIVITIES

> ✏ **You will need:**
> **paper, colouring pens/crayons/watercolour paints.**

1. Maybe you are now feeling inspired to write a little love poem starting with 'Love is when you…'. Any decoration will do nicely to complete your writing.

2. Another idea is to try and remember or find other sayings about the heart and then write them down under the title 'Heart exercise'. To make it look pleasing to the eye you could decorate this page with love symbols.

3. Starting today, you could keep a diary about situations when you have been aware of your heartbeat. Illustrations may help to express your ideas.

4. How about asking your parents and siblings when they have felt the rhythm of their heartbeat change and whether you can feel it.

Over the next week, really observe what is happening with your heart – during P.E. lessons, when you run to catch the bus, when you are very happy. I would also like you to have a close look at what happens when you are feeling nervous, anxious or afraid of something. Quietly say the heart magic words several times to yourself. Does anything change?

WEEK 5: 'STOMACH'

The stomach magic words are…

'My stomach is wonderfully warm'.

Read the new magic words out loud before you add this one onto the previous ones.

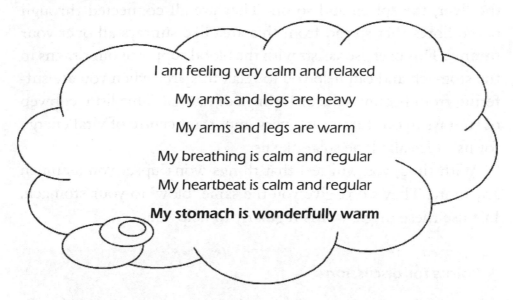

I am feeling very calm and relaxed

My arms and legs are heavy

My arms and legs are warm

My breathing is calm and regular

My heartbeat is calm and regular

My stomach is wonderfully warm

What happens? In this exercise you have to imagine a wonderful feeling warming up your stomach. It could be like a big warm soft wave or long sunrays reaching every little part of your stomach, giving you a magical sensation. You can give them a warm colour, maybe yellow or orange.

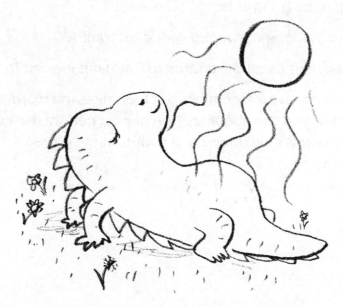

What's the purpose? In a soft area in your tummy, tucked away safely, are a lot of your important organs: the intestines or bowels, the liver, the spleen and so on. They are all connected through nerve fibres that spread from this area like sunrays all over your tummy. This exercise assists with the blood supply of our organs in the stomach and can help you to relax this area when you are suffering from tummy ache or feelings of nausea. This little cobweb of sunrays in our tummy is a very important centre of vital energy for us. It is called the solar plexus.

With time, you will feel that things won't upset you as much any more. They won't give you the same 'blow' to your stomach. Just use these magic words regularly to help you.

Points for discussion

- What should you not do before practising the relaxation magic words? If you are finding it difficult to relax your stomach it can be because you've eaten too much before doing this exercise and your stomach is full. It is advisable to practise before having eaten. A light snack is a good idea to prevent you from being really hungry as that is not good either.

- Have you ever massaged your own tummy?

- What does it feel like afterwards? What is it good for?

- If you do give it a gentle rub, it feels nice and warm and relaxed and the abdominal circulation gets increased. This means more blood is in your tummy to keep it warm.

WARM-UP ACTIVITIES

> ✏ **You will need: a hot water bottle or a warm aroma cushion or a pair of warm hands.**

1. If you are at home

   In preparation for this exercise, you could put a hot water bottle on your stomach, just above your belly button to help you create a feeling of warmth in this area. Some families have little aroma cushions that can be warmed up in the microwave or the oven. That is another alternative to understand what feeling this fifth relaxation exercise is meant to create in you.

2. If you are not at home or at school

   You could warm up your hands by massaging them and then put your hands onto your friend's stomach so they experience a nice feeling of warmth. This will help you to understand the fifth magic words and what it is supposed to feel like.

You can now start the stomach exercise, saying all the magic words three to six times quietly in your mind or listening to the story being read to you. Lie down/sit down feeling the warmth in the soft area of your stomach as if there is a little sun inside you. Your stomach is beautifully warm. Don't forget to 'close' the exercise properly at the end unless this is bedtime for you.

THE STOMACH STORY

The Hidden Beach

You are lying on a soft blanket on the floor and you are starting to relax. You are taking a deep breath in mhh...and let all the air out again...that's right, very good...you are beginning to *feel very calm and relaxed...* The big blue bubble sweeps you up and off you fly out of the room into the clear nothingness. You can see a few tiny white clouds dotted around and occasionally they bump into the bubble and make you wriggle your head a little bit...you smile.

You have been flying for a while when the bubble takes you to a tiny little beach, hidden away in amongst pink, towering rocks... It is absolutely stunning. You walk along in the soft, white sand, the sun is shining and reflected in the shades of blue and turquoise of the wide ocean water. In the distance you can see young dolphins jumping and playing about. They are really enjoying themselves. In fact, it's a whole family of dolphins. Then you notice Deeno who is building a sandcastle and you help him to decorate it with the pretty shells that you found on your walk. It has turned into a majestic castle. You decide to go for a little swim.

The water is lovely and warm and quite shallow. After lots of swimming and playing around in the water with Deeno you decide to lie down...*your arms and legs feel really heavy* from building that sandcastle and ...*your arms and legs feel nice and warm* after playing around in the tiny waves in the warm water. You are beginning to feel sleepy...*your breathing is calm and regular* like the gentle crashing of the waves in the ocean and you can feel your heart beating very softly...*your heartbeat is calm and regular...* The sun is shining bright, warming your relaxed body and sending you new energy and warm comforting rays of sunshine onto your tummy...*your stomach is wonderfully warm.* It's as if a warm wave is slowly flooding your stomach, giving you a beautiful feeling inside. Enjoy that feeling just a little bit longer...that's it...you are very safe at this little beach surrounded by the pink rocks...your stomach is relaxing more with every wave of warmth that is flowing through you...there is no place where you'd rather be.

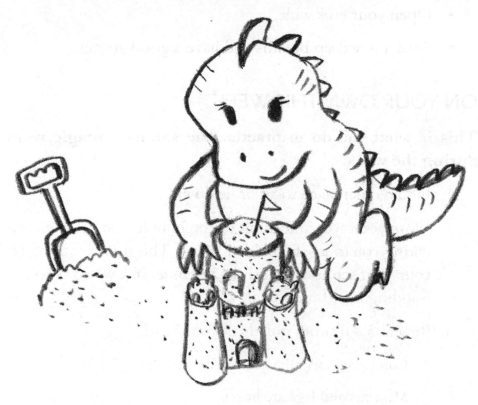

[PAUSE]

Then you sit up and see the blue bubble emerging. One more time, you watch the playful dolphins in the distance, hear their happy sounds and the splashing of water. You take a good look around the beautiful little beach and, together, you and Deeno climb into the bubble, leaving this wonderful haven of peace and happiness behind you. You are feeling deeply relaxed and content. This is an amazing place which you can choose to go back to in your mind at any time during the week to come and relax yourself.

In a few minutes, I would like you to get ready to 'close' the exercise:

- Make a strong fist with both hands.

- Bend/flex your elbows sharply several times.

- Open your eyes wide.

- Take a few deep breaths and have a good stretch.

ON YOUR OWN THIS WEEK

This is what you do to practise the stomach magic words during the week.

1. Find a quiet place to sit or lie down.

2. Close your eyes and think of the bubble coming your way, taking you to a safe, hidden beach. The sun is shining and your stomach is wonderfully warm as if a warm wave was flooding it with new energy.

3. Repeat 3 – 6 times quietly in your head:

    I am feeling very calm and relaxed

    My arms and legs are heavy

    My arms and legs are warm

    My breathing is calm and regular

    My heartbeat is calm and regular

    My stomach is wonderfully warm

4. Concentrate on feeling the warmth in your stomach.

5. Don't forget to close the exercise at the end unless it is bedtime.

FOLLOW-UP ACTIVITIES

✐ **You will need:**
paper, colouring pens or crayons or watercolour
paints.

Take some paper, colouring pens, crayons or watercolour paints and a paint brush and do the following:

- Draw a picture of a beautiful beach, the sea, the dolphins and the sun that warmed your stomach and the little cobweb of sunrays inside you.

- Maybe you feel like drawing that powerful sun and the sunrays. You can use the most magical colour combinations for this picture. I am sure it will look fantastic.

- Alternatively, you might want to write a little poem about the warmth and strength of the sun. Think about the importance of the sun for so many living creatures on earth; the flowers, trees, shrubs, birds, other animals, the farmers and their fields of wheat, rye, vegetables and so on. Let your imagination take you where you will find the rays of the sun... They will have to be positive images in order to help you with this exercise.

WEEK 6: 'FOREHEAD'

The forehead magic words are...

'My forehead is nice and cool'.

Read the important note below, and the new magic words and add them onto last week's.

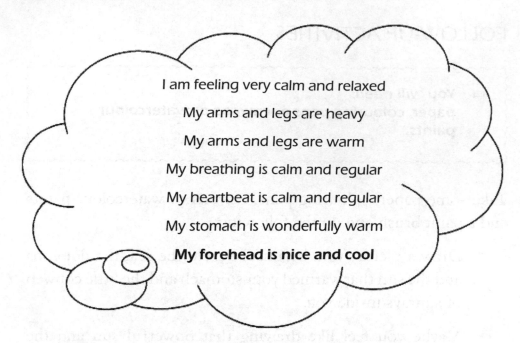

I am feeling very calm and relaxed

My arms and legs are heavy

My arms and legs are warm

My breathing is calm and regular

My heartbeat is calm and regular

My stomach is wonderfully warm

My forehead is nice and cool

Important note:

Here you go; you've arrived at the last exercise. Well done for sticking with it this far. This is the only exercise in the classic Autogenic relaxation technique that asks you to imagine a pleasant feeling of coolness. Cooling the forehead alongside warming the body has been proven to have a calming effect on you. You should only learn this new exercise once you have really mastered the others. CAREFUL: This exercise should not be done at bedtime. It gives you new energy and concentration and does not help you to fall asleep.

What happens? In this exercise, it is important that you imagine a very pleasant coolness of your forehead. It could for example be the cooling hand of a loving person, or a refreshing summer breeze. You know how it feels when you have a temperature and a cold flannel is put on your forehead, which is very pleasant and a great relief. That is exactly the sensation this exercise is meant to create in you.

What's the purpose? To stay cool-headed! The head is the only area in which warmth is not particularly pleasant. With a warm head you cannot concentrate very well, you cannot 'get it all into your head'. So when you feel tired and are trying to do your home-work just close your eyes, say these magic words several times quietly to yourself and you will see that the strong image of a cool breeze on your forehead will help you to clear your head and to work at full speed again. With time and practice, you will chill out more, get fewer headaches and be less of a hot-headed person.

Points for discussion

What gives you a pleasant feeling of having a clear head?

- Ever tried a strong mint? What does it do to your nose and forehead?

- Have you ever been on a flying carpet? Where could it take you? How would it feel flying through the air?

- Have you ever been out on a lovely summer's day with a pleasant cool breeze? How does that feel?

WARM-UP ACTIVITIES

✏ **No equipment needed, just a little space to move around, perhaps some happy music and some pieces of paper acting as leaves.**

A windy Autumn day – acting out an autumn scene – be dramatic, play and improvise:

Imagine, it's a windy Autumn day and you are outside, playing in a big country park. You are running around, enjoying the noise of the leaves as you are rushing through them, blowing them into the air with your hands and feet. It is so much fun to see them flying around. Autumn is a fantastic time of year.

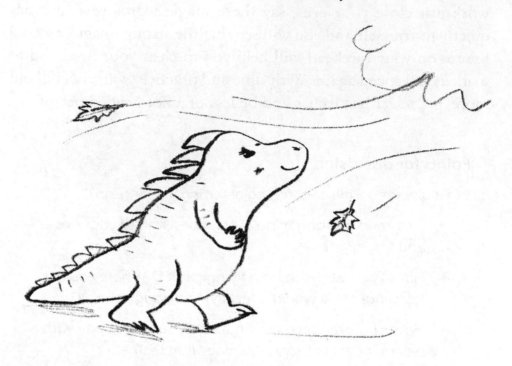

After a while you are getting quite hot and a little tired. You find yourself a nice little place, you sit down to relax for a while and you suddenly feel a wonderful soft, cold stone next to you.

You pick up the stone and put it onto your forehead. It feels so pleasant and cool and you have the most wonderful feeling…the coolness of this stone is magical…all the tiredness disappears… you are enjoying the pleasant coolness of your forehead, how it spreads everywhere in your head.

You feel ready to go back, you say good-bye to the stone and full of energy and happiness you leave the park and go home and join your family for dinner.

You can now start the forehead exercise, saying all the magic words three to six times quietly in your mind. Lie or sit down, feeling the pleasant coolness of your forehead whilst the rest of your body is nice and warm. *Remember, don't do the forehead exercise at bedtime.*

THE FOREHEAD STORY

Magic on a Mountain Meadow

Imagine you are on holiday in the country. It is a warm sunny day and it's Autumn. This is a beautiful season with all the trees changing colour and the crunchy sound of walking over crisp leaves on the ground is unique to this time of the year. The sky is blue, not a cloud on the horizon. You breathe in the fresh air and *you are feeling very calm and relaxed.* You are very happy to be outdoors and you look up at the mountain that you can see in the distance; it is majestic, so strong and upright. You really like that mountain and, as you are contemplating what to do, Deeno, your friend the dinosaur, comes along and says: 'Hello! Do you want to climb that mountain with me today?' 'That's a great idea,' you hear yourself saying and off you go. You find a winding path and follow it around and around the mountain... Higher and higher. You are both working quite hard at getting up that mountain but the views are stunning. Deeno keeps telling you little jokes that make you laugh and, before you know it, you arrive at the top. It's fantastic; you've come to a mountain meadow, with lush green grass and big old trees. It's fairly windy up here. Walking is so much fun as you can really bend forward and the wind carries you. After a while you are getting tired and so you find yourself a nice little place. You sit down to relax for a while and make yourself comfortable. *Your arms and legs feel really heavy* and after having walked all the way up that mountain your *arms and legs feel really warm.* You can feel your blood circulating like a rushing river inside your body *making you feel so warm everywhere.*

As you are resting for a while under this lovely old tree your *breathing is becoming calm and regular.* Deeno is lying very close to you, so close that you can feel that he has fallen asleep because his

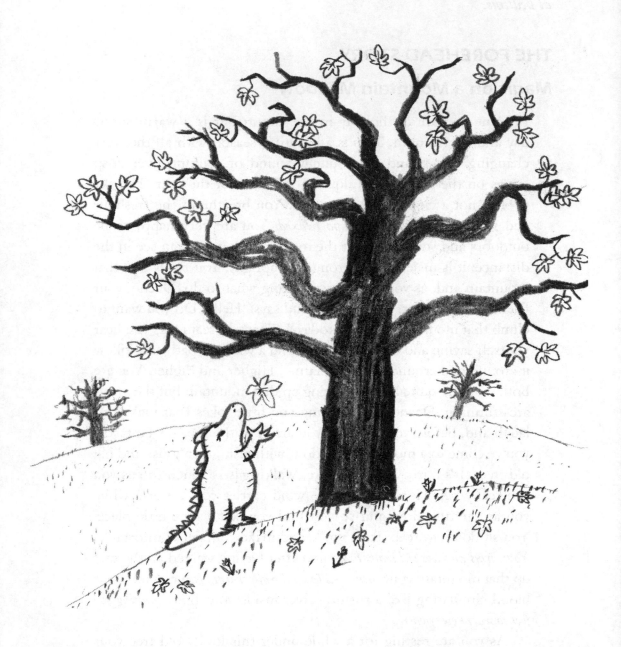

heartbeat is so calm and regular. As you are feeling Deeno's heart-beat being so calm and regular *your own heartbeat is getting very calm and regular.* And as you are resting there, the sun is shining onto your stomach, making *it wonderfully warm. Your stomach is wonderfully warm.* You enjoy watching the Autumn leaves as they are flying past you doing the most wonderful acrobatics in the air until one very special leaf lands right next to you. 'Hello,' it whispers to you, 'I am the magic leaf and, if you want, I can do magic for you!' … You smile, stretch out on the soft dry ground and close your eyes… you take that beautiful magic colourful leaf and for a few minutes place it *onto your forehead… It feels so pleasant and cool* and you have the most wonderful feeling…the coolness of this leaf is magical…all the tiredness disappears, you are enjoying the pleasant coolness of your forehead, how it spreads everywhere in your head…you are feeling totally refreshed, relaxed and happy as if coming back from a long holiday. As you are flying back in the big blue bubble you and Deeno can feel the pleasant coolness on your forehead one more time. Then it's time to say good-bye to each other.

- Make a strong fist with both hands.

- Bend/flex your elbows sharply several times.

- Open your eyes wide.

- Take a few deep breaths and have a good stretch.

ON YOUR OWN THIS WEEK

This is what you do to practise the forehead magic words during the week.

1. Find a quiet place to sit or lie down.

2. Close your eyes and think of the bubble coming your way, taking you to a windy mountain meadow with lots of leaves dancing about. One leaf is on your forehead, giving you

a very pleasant feeling of coolness. Feel how your head is flooded with clarity and concentration.

3. Repeat three to six times quietly in your head:

> I am feeling very calm and relaxed
>
> My arms and legs are heavy
>
> My arms and legs are warm
>
> My breathing is calm and regular
>
> My heartbeat is calm and regular
>
> My stomach is wonderfully warm
>
> **My forehead is nice and cool**

4. Concentrate on feeling the coolness of your forehead.

Remember, don't do this exercise at bedtime.

FOLLOW-UP ACTIVITIES

Choose one or several activities – they will be great fun and will help you to remember the forehead magic words.

✏ **You will need:**

1. **paper, colouring pens/crayons/watercolour paints, brushes**

2. **a collection of various leaves from the garden or park**

3. **cardboard, glue stick, wooden sticks/string, scissors**

4. **happy, fast music, some space for dancing and possibly light material or an old bed sheet.**

1. *Your magic Autumn leaf*: Try to find some paper, colouring pens, crayons or watercolour paints and a paint brush and draw or paint your magic Autumn leaf exactly the way you remember it so that you can always look at it and remind yourself how good that felt on your forehead.

2. *A colourful collage*: Go into the garden or the park and collect as many leaves as you can find and create a colourful collage.

3. *A garden scene*: Create a whole Autumn forest or garden scene with leaves and bushes, trees, and lots of wind. There are wonderful things you can find in the woods that the wind has brought down from the trees so you can pick them up, take them home in a little bag and use them for a creative nature picture.

4. *Creating a mobile*: It is good fun to create a mobile with leaves. Choose about five or seven leaves or draw them, cut out their shapes in cardboard and stick these onto the leaves to make them stronger and heavier. Then make a hole in each one, get some string and thin wooden sticks (the ones used for kebabs) and make it into a lovely mobile. How about putting it up just over your bed?

5. *The leaves' dance*: Put on some happy music and imagine that you are a leaf outside on a windy day. There is a big white cloud that is blowing you in all directions. You are running around, turning, rolling over on the floor, lying down for a while until the wind picks you up again. You are twirling around like a spinning top. If a friend or one of your siblings wants to play with you, you could ask for an old bed sheet. One of you pretends to be the wind running behind you, blowing and blowing... In the summer, it is great to do this outside. You'll see how this makes you feel very energetic and cheerful.

CREATING YOUR OWN MAGIC WORDS

Magic words for power and strength

Once you have come as far as this page of the book, you are ready to go up a level in your relaxation training to become a true expert. However, you should only ever start on this chapter once you have properly mastered all the magic words in the previous chapter! The idea is to add these special magic words onto the basic magic words that you have learnt during the past six weeks.

In this chapter you are going to learn how to make up your own magic words, which, repeated daily, will make you feel very confident in the most nerve-racking situations. It is like programming yourself with new computer game software.

First of all, you will have to teach your body your chosen magic words just like you did with the six basic magic words from the Autogenic exercises. After a few weeks of practice your body will be programmed to react to it, just like it learnt to react to the six magic words.

Magic words are also called 'positive affirmations' and they will help you to overcome fear and nervousness. They will make you strong and calm in any situation.

The idea is to make up words for each situation which presents a challenge to you. For example, if you find it hard to concentrate and get your thoughts together to do your homework or revise for a test, or even during a test, the following magic words might be just right for you:

Concentration is a breeze - I do it with ease!

or

My inner light is shining bright and helps me to get it right!

or

I can concentrate and that's really great!

Thinking up your magic words

There are lots of different ways of thinking up magic words. The main thing is that they must sound right and work for you. The secret is that when you say the words to yourself they must make you feel really good and positive. Otherwise, they are not magic for you. What you must ensure is that magic words never go together with the words no, don't, isn't, can't or any negative words like fear, pain, problem, etc. They are purely encouraging and have to put you in a very confident, positive mood.

If the magic words rhyme they are easier to remember, but they also work as short snappy sentences. A good way to start is *'I can...'* or *'I am...'* or *'I feel...'*. I will give you a few magic word combinations to get the idea. However, you need to decide which ones are important and can be helpful for you. The words must come naturally and sound right to you.

Some examples of magic words

- I feel calm and warm inside!

- To be at rest is best!

- I can be calm!

- I'm taking my time – that's fine!

- My time is mine!

- I can go to any length with strength!

- I can see the light and I am doing it right!

- Focus means success – at school and in sports.

- Concentration through relaxation is the happiness equation!

- I can hear, so it's clear!

What you think of most is what you get most

Whatever wc focus on and believe about ourselves becomes a reality for us. If you think you are no good, you won't be! If, on the other hand you think you can do it and you put as much practice into something as you can, you will do it! So, it is incredibly important to have fantastic beliefs about who we are and what we can achieve and do in life. Our bodies will listen to our thoughts and act accordingly. If you do kind and generous things like praising or helping a friend regularly, and you tell yourself every day and with total conviction how wonderful and special you are, you will come to believe it.

Twenty-one days for the magic to work

You can use these magic words in any situation in the future. Twenty-one days are usually needed for the message to sink in and for your body to absorb it. For example, three weeks before a challenging situation or an important event you can start saying the magic words in your mind, at the end of your magic words practice, early in the morning or at night just before falling asleep. With your eyes closed, really concentrate on imagining yourself in that nerve-racking situation in the future. See how you stand, what you wear, what you are saying, how confident you feel, smiling and holding yourself. Feel what it is like to be truly confident, calm and positive before, during and after the event. It may help to think of another event in the past which you mastered really well and feel good about and link this feeling to the challenging situation ahead of you. Make sure your out-breath is very long and keep hold of that strong, positive calm feeling inside. Keep on saying your magic words, totally feeling, seeing, hearing and believing in your ability to master whatever situation it is.

What are particularly challenging situations for you? What are your ideas for magic words that will help you? This cloud is for you to fill with **your magic words**:

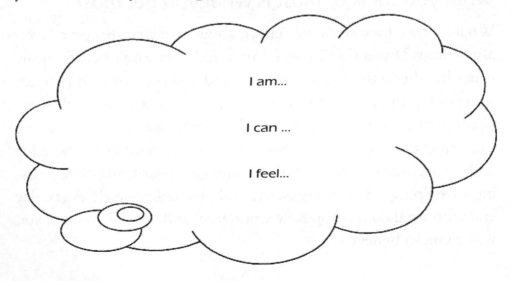

I am...

I can ...

I feel...

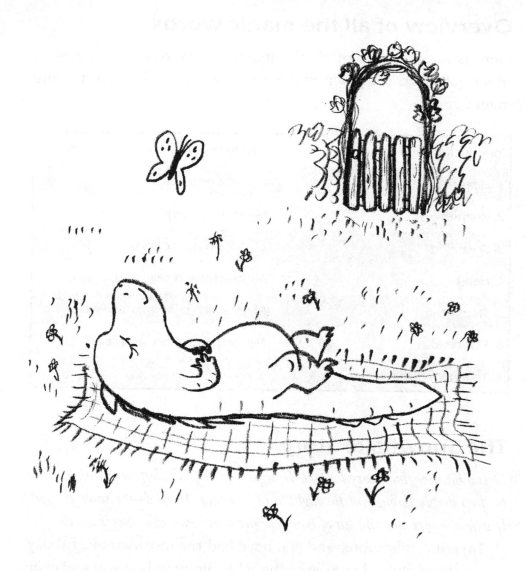

In the beginning, it is best to use your chosen magic words along with the other six weeks of magic words you have just learnt, maybe after the stomach or the forehead magic words. You will feel when the moment has come to use your magic words on their own when you need them; for example just before a test when sitting at school, feeling worried, or at night when you wake up and cannot sleep. They are amazingly powerful.

Overview of all the magic words

Here is an overview of all the magic words you have learnt in this book. Add your own words to the end, and have fun doing magic!

Introduction with Calmness	I am feeling very calm and relaxed
1. Heaviness	My arms and legs are heavy
2. Warmth	My arms and legs are warm
3. Breathing	My breathing is calm and regular
4. Heart	My heartbeat is calm and regular
5. Stomach	My stomach is wonderfully warm
6. Forehead	My forehead is nice and cool
7. Your own magic words...	. . . .

The Snowflake Story

Deeno has one final story for you. It helps him to fall asleep very quickly and to sleep deeply throughout the night, and he hopes it will do the same for you. It will also give you an idea of how you might use your own magic words.

Imagine, it is winter and you have had the most wonderful day out in the snow and now, at night, when lying in bed you feel ever so good. You remember all the children's high-spirited, boisterous laughter, meeting your friends and seeing the happy faces of other Mums, Dads, children and dogs playing in the cold, white snowy park. You remember having friendly snow fights, building big burly snowmen and funny snow women in pink ballet skirts and spending hours making wonderful white creatures with imaginative decorations and colourful outfits. It was such a fun day.

You are lying in bed and your eye-lids are starting to feel very heavy, they are feeling very heavy and as you are lying there so comfortably snuggled up in bed, you remember your relaxation and your magic words …You concentrate on your breathing and then the big blue bubble embraces you and takes you to a far away place. Deeno is sitting in the bubble, smiling away. It is always great to be with Deeno. He gives you the thumbs up 'OK' sign and you are starting to feel *very calm and relaxed*, especially after all the running around in the snow today.

You are breathing in … and out….. , very calmly, breathing in……and out…..and you are starting to feel *very calm and relaxed* all over, in every part of your body. [PAUSE]

After a while, you start to feel a very *comforting heaviness in your arms and legs, the muscles around your eyes, your jaw, your neck and shoulders, all feel nice and heavy and then slowly this heaviness spreads all over your body making you very calm and relaxed.* You can feel your blood travelling much more evenly and freely throughout your body, and *your arms and legs feel pleasantly warm all over. Your arms and legs feel pleasantly warm all over.* It is warm and so comfortable in the bubble and there is no place you'd rather be right now.

Then, the bubble lands. It lands in a soft, white silent place, the place where the snowflakes live. You and Deeno are in the middle of a fairy tale winter dream [PAUSE]

Everything is white in front of you. As far as you can see, all is white and so peaceful. You see snowflakes dancing so gracefully, drawing the most amazing patterns in the sky – you can see ice flowers, ice trees, ice fairies and ice dwarfs quietly sipping a hot white chocolate drink with happy glowing faces. Further back you can see a big calm polar bear skating on a frozen lake, he is gently gliding over the ice in figures of eight with a shy family of deer and a little Robin watching with admiration from a distance on the safe shore.

Deeno's *breathing is calm and regular, his chest is going gently up…and down…up and down…and so is yours. Your breathing is calm and regular. It feels very relaxing and soothing.* [PAUSE] – *You can also feel Deeno's heartbeat beautifully calm and regular next to you and it feels very calming, very calming and after a few minutes, your heartbeat is also beautifully calm and regular, calm and regular.* There is nothing you have to do right now, just feel the wonderful relaxing, calm, regular beating of your own heart.

You are lying in the bubble and it is so peaceful to see this white scenery from the warm, cosy blue bubble full of cushions and blankets. You are feeling very safe and calm from deep within. *Your stomach is beginning to feel lovely and warm, lovely and warm,* giving you new energy for the coming day. [PAUSE] – Then, you notice one particularly beautiful snowflake dancing right in front of you, her moves are a delight, so soft, elegant, skilful and yet very calm. It's as if she is smiling at you and Deeno and then you hear her singing in the most pure and lovely, rhythmic voice 'As soon as I close my eyes, I go drifting off asleep'. *'As soon as I close my eyes, I go drifting off asleep'. 'As soon as I close my eyes, I go drifting off asleep'.*…you are quietly repeating those magic words in your mind [PAUSE]. You are quietly repeating those magic words in your mind until you can no longer see or hear anything. Deeno has already fallen asleep and you follow shortly into this deep, sweet sleep. [PAUSE] - And the next morning, when you wake up you feel totally happy, energetic and calmly confident, knowing that in your mind, you can always go back to this wonderful, safe, magic place.

Part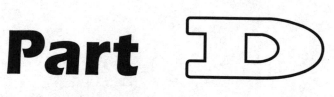

Resources

Further reading

Relaxation for children

My trainers, Dr. Patricia Aden, Sabine Seyffert and Claudia Reeker-Lange whose publications are to be found in German, have been successfully using Autogenics with children and adults for over ten years and are experts in the field of relaxation and Autogenics.

As far as I am aware, however, there are currently no publications other than this one in English on using Autogenics with children. However, a number of authors have approached the subject of children's relaxation from other angles.

Books

Pearson, M. (2004) *Emotional Healing and Self-Esteem: Inner-life Skills of Relaxation, Visualisation and Meditation for Children and Adolescents.* London: Jessica Kingsley Publishers.

Fontana, D. and Slack, I. *Teaching Meditation to Children.* London: Element Books.

Berschma, D. and Visscher, M. (2003) *Yoga Games for Children.* USA: Alameda CA: Hunter House Inc.

Rozen, D. *Meditating With Children.* London: Tree Press.

Seligman, M. (2007) *The Optimistic Child: A Proven Program to Safeguard Children against Depression and Build Lifelong Resilience.* US Imports.

Audio CDs

Kerr, C. has published meditation CDs for children available from www.hypnosi-saudio.com and Divinity Publishing Ltd.

Lite, L. has published CDs on relaxation for children which you can find under www.LiteBooks.net

Viegas, M. has published mediation CDs for toddlers and children available from www.relaxkids.com

Autogenics for adults

Schultz, J.L. with Luthe, W. (1969 and 1970) *Autogenic Therapy Vols 1-4*. New York: Grune & Stratton. (Written by the founder of the technique.)

Bird, J. with Pinch, C. (2002) *Autogenic Therapy*. Dublin: Newleaf.

Linden, W. (1990) *Autogenic Training: A Clinical Guide*. New York: The Guilford Press.

On parenting

Bandura, A. (1989) 'Social cognitive theories.' In R. Vasta (ed.) *Annals of Child Development, 6. Six Theories of Child Development* (pp.1–60). Greenwich, CT: Jai Press.

Bandura, A. and Walters, R.H. (1959) *Adolescent Aggression; a Study of the Influence of Child-Training Practices and Family Interrelationships*. New York: Ronald Press.

Boakes, R. (1984) *From Darwin to Behaviourism*. Cambridge: Cambridge University Press.

Chacham, M. (2008) *How to Calm a Challenging Child*. London: Foulsham.

Covey, S.R. (1999) *The 7 Habits of Highly Effective Families*. London: Simon & Schuster.

Palmer, S. (2007) *Detoxing Childhood*. London: Orion Publishing.

Sunderland, M. (2006) *What Every Parent Needs to Know*. London: Dorling Kindersley. (In its first edition it was called *The Science of Parenting*.)

Interesting articles

Lohaus, A., KleinHeßling, J. and Shebar, S. (1997) 'Stress management for elementary school children: A comparative evaluation of different approaches.' *European Review of Applied Psychology, 47*, 157–161.

Lohaus, A. and KleinHeßling, J. (2000) 'Coping in childhood: A comparative evaluation of different relaxation techniques.' *Anxiety, Stress, and Coping, 13*, 187–211.

Lohaus, A., KleinHeßling, J., Vögele, C. and KuhnHenninghausen, C. (2001) 'Relaxation in children: Effects on physiological measures.' *British Journal of Health Psychology, 6*, 197–206.

Goldbeck, L. and Schmid, K. (2003) 'Effectiveness of Autogenic relaxation training on children and adolescents with behavioral and emotional problems.' *Journal of the American Academy of Child & Adolescent Psychiatry, 42*(9), 1046–1054 http://findarticles.com/p/articles/mi_qa4087/is_/ai_n9353086

Mulgannon, T. (Oct.1998) 'Relaxation on demand – stress management advice from the book *Autogenic Training: a Clinical Guide* by psychology professor Wolfgang Linden. *Men's Fitness.* http://findarticles.com/p/articles/mi_m1608/is_/ai_21148333?tag=artBody;coll

Useful websites

On parenting

www.familyeducation.com – offers some interesting ideas on relaxation for children and their families.

www.fathersdirect.com – to give information on fatherhood.

www.mumsnet.com – post your parenting questions, make new connections.

www.sleepforkids.org – offers information on sleep.

www.raisingkids.co.uk – general advice.

www.bbc.co.uk/parenting – offering varied advice for your family life.

www.parentlineplus.org.uk – offering help with bullying.

Other useful sites

www.chalkface.com – useful advice for teachers.

www.aap.org – good recommended reading section.

www.psychosomatic.org – website of the American Psychosomatic Society.

www.nccam.nih.gov – information on complementary and alternative medicine.